Souleymane TANGARA

Medical thesis

Souleymane TANGARA

Medical thesis

Epidemioclinics and therapeutics of thoracic and vascular pathologies at the André FESTOC center of theCHU-ME of Bamako

Imprint

Any brand names and product names mentioned in this book are subject to trademark, brand or patent protection and are trademarks or registered trademarks of their respective holders. The use of brand names, product names, common names, trade names, product descriptions etc. even without a particular marking in this work is in no way to be construed to mean that such names may be regarded as unrestricted in respect of trademark and brand protection legislation and could thus be used by anyone.

Cover image: www.ingimage.com

This book is a translation from the original published under ISBN 978-620-6-72347-9.

Publisher:
Sciencia Scripts
is a trademark of
Dodo Books Indian Ocean Ltd. and OmniScriptum S.R.L publishing group

120 High Road, East Finchley, London, N2 9ED, United Kingdom
Str. Armeneasca 28/1, office 1, Chisinau MD-2012, Republic of Moldova, Europe
Printed at: see last page
ISBN: 978-620-8-20740-3

Contents

DEDICATIONS AND THANKS

DEDICACES

I love this work

A ALLAH

The omniscient, the omnipotent, the Creator of heaven and earth, the All-Merciful, the Most-Merciful, the One who is the basis of everything, the One who gave me courage and luck during these long years of study. May Your will be done Lord, and I pray that your presence will continue throughout my medical practice.

To my Father Sina TANGARA

For all the moments of attention, sacrifice and dedication I have enjoyed with you. You instilled in us a strong sense of responsibility and dignity, tolerance, rigour, a job well done, modesty, respect, honour and perseverance - in short, all the qualities that a man should acquire. I cannot find the words to express how proud I am to be your son. May you find, Father, in this modest work, a real reason for satisfaction. May ALLAH grant you a long life in good health so that you can see us succeed and benefit from your blessings.

To my Mother Aminata DEMBELE

Dear mother, an exemplary educator, you never tired of accepting and loving others with all their differences; you cultivated in us the virtues of tolerance and love of neighbour against a background of tenderness and affection. Please find here, dear mother, the expression of our deep gratitude and unfailing love. You put a lot of effort into my success. Your philosophy of life is a benchmark for all of us in terms of courage, generosity and simplicity. Thanks to your sacrifices and dedication, your son has become a doctor. May God the Almighty bless you abundantly and keep you by our side for as long as possible so that we can continue to benefit from your advice and your love.

THANKS :

"Whatever the value of the moment given to a man, there is only one word to express the gratitude inspired by generosity, and that word is THANK YOU", said our compatriot the late Amadou Hampate Ba, may his soul rest in peace, in his work entitled L'Etrange destin de Wangrin (The Strange Destiny of Wangrin).

Thank you, thank you to all those who supported me during those long years of study, because where I come from, the past is not forgotten.

TRIBUTES TO THE MEMBERS OF THE JURY

TO OUR MASTER PRESIDENT OF THE JURY

Professor Seydou TOGO

- Specialist in Thoracic and Cardiovascular Surgery;
- Professor of Thoracic and Cardiovascular Surgery at the FMOS;
- Hospital practitioner at I'hopital du Mali ;
- Founding member of the Society of Thoracic and Cardiovascular Surgery of Mali.

Dear Master

You have done us the great honour of agreeing to chair our thesis jury. The privilege of having as a teacher a man of science as modest and rigorous as you is for us a legacy of life. Your availability enabled us to carry out this work with the minimum of difficulty. Your great humanity and sense of justice impressed us. Your scientific and social values and your personality are for us an ideal of excellence and wisdom.

TO OUR MASTER AND JUDGE

Professor Brehima BENGALY

- Associate Professor of General Surgery at the Faculty of Medicine and Odontostomatology /USTTB
- Hospital practitioner at CHU point G
- Master in pedagogy
- Member of the Mali Surgery Society
- Medical epidemiologist.

Dear Master

We are delighted and honoured that you have spontaneously agreed to judge this thesis. Your competence and your deep sense of humanity are known to all. Your criticisms, suggestions and encouragement will be of capital importance in improving the quality of this work. Please find here the expression of our most distinguished consideration.

TO OUR MASTER AND JUDGE

Doctor BABA IBRAHIMA DIARRA

- Senior Research Fellow in Cardiovascular Surgery CNRST
- Head of Department of Thoracic and Cardiovascular Surgery at the Andre FESTOC Centre at the Mere - Enfant "le Luxembourg" Hospital in Bamako.
- Thoracic and cardiovascular surgeon at the Andre FESTOC centre at the Mere - Enfant "Luxembourg" hospital in Bamako.
- Masters in morphological and clinical anatomy at UCAD, Dakar

Dear Master

You have done us an immense honour by accepting us into your department. We would like to thank you most sincerely for agreeing to serve on this noble jury. We are honoured by your presence. We have had the privilege of benefiting from your high-quality teaching. Your simplicity, your teaching skills and your scientific mind make you a master admired and respected by all. May this work express, dear master, all our esteem, our deep gratitude and our complete confidence. Please find here the expression of our deepest respect.

TO OUR MASTER AND CO - THESIS DIRECTOR

Doctor Modibo Doumbia

- **Senior research fellow in cardiovascular surgery at the CNRST**
- **Representative of the Minister for Health**
- **President of the Bamako District Medical Association**
- **Thoracic and cardiovascular surgeon at the Andre FESTOC Centre at the Mere - Enfant "Luxembourg" Hospital in Bamako**
- **Masters in morphological and clinical anatomy at UCAD, Dakar**
- **Inter-university diploma in medical informatics Dear Master**

We would like to take this opportunity to express our great esteem and admiration for you. Throughout this work, we have appreciated your great human and scientific qualities, your teaching, your strong sense of responsibility, your approachability and, above all, your rigour in your work. Dear Master, you have instilled in us team spirit, endurance, perseverance, a job well done and, above all, patience. May ALLAH grant you a long life in good health and full of success in your projects.

TO OUR MASTER AND THESIS DIRECTOR

Professor Birama TOGOLA

- **Full Professor of General Surgery**
- **Specialist in Thoracic and Cardiovascular Surgery**
- **Inter-university diploma in pedagogy and communication science**
- **University diploma in peripheral vascular endo**
- **Fellow of the West African College of Surgeons (WACS)**
- **Member of the Malian Surgery Society (SOCHIMA)**
- **Member of the Malian Society of Thoracic and Cardiovascular Surgery (SOTCAV)**
- **Hospital practitioner at the CHU du point "G".**

Dear Master

You have done us a great honour by agreeing to entrust us with this work. We would like to thank you for your patience, your availability, your encouragement and your valuable advice in carrying out this work. Your competence, dynamism and rigour have aroused in us great admiration and deep respect. Your professional and human qualities serve as an example to us all. Please accept the expression of my deepest gratitude and respect.

I- Introduction

Thoracic and vascular surgery is the academic discipline of medicine encompassing the techniques and methods of prevention, diagnosis and surgical treatment of congenital or acquired thoracic and vascular disorders [1].

This дёГтя^и can in some cases be ëtended to affections of the frontiëres of the thorax (neck, breast and diaphragm).

Their spëcificitë is that they depend on the vital organs to which they are intëressed and the technological environment necessary for their practice.

In the West, thoracic pathologies of infectious origin were by far the most frequent, but with industrialization and modernization, cancerous pathologies now occupy first place [2].

In France, lung cancer was the 3rd most common cancer, with 52,777 new cases diagnosed in 2023 [3].

In developing countries, particularly in Africa, surgical thoracic pathologies are still dominated by infectious diseases [4].

In West Africa, several studies have been carried out on vascular pathologies. According to Konin C et al [6] in 2015 in Cote d'Ivoire the prevalence of chronic venous insufficiency of the lower limbs was 60.4%. For Haounou F et al [7] in 2016 in Benin DVT ëtait localisëe aux membres infërieurs chez 51,3% des patients. For James Didier L et al [8] in 2018 in Niger, the rare occurrence of arterial hypertension was due to under-diagnosis and a lack of specialists.

The practice of thoracic and vascular surgery in Mali dates back to the early years of independence. The first thoracotomy in Mali was performed by Professor **Mamadou Dembele in 1963 [9]**. In **1983**, Professors AK **Koumare** and **Alain Decloche** performed the first open-heart commissurotomy.

In Mali, according to Nganmeni Ignace [9] in 2006, surgical thoracic pathologies accounted for 13.03% of hospitalisations in the "A" surgery department at the CHU du Point "G". According to Guindo I O [10] in 2013, purulent pleurisy represented 1.95% of pyothoraxes in the pneumology department at the CHU Point "G".

Thoracic and vascular surgery is a fast-growing speciality thanks to new technologies, and is currently subdivided into several sub-specialities, in particular pleuropulmonary, chest wall and peripheral vascular surgery.

In 2011, a thoracic and vascular surgery department was set up at **the Mali Hospital** for the first time in order to improve care for these conditions. In view of the increased need for thoracic and vascular surgery care and the return from training of certain specialists, a thoracic and cardiovascular surgery reference centre called **the "Andre FESTOC centre"** was created in September 2018 at the **CHU mere-enfant le Luxembourg in BAMAKO** thanks to l'ONG chaine de l'espoir. The centre is a sub-regional reference for the diagnostic and therapeutic management of thoracic and vascular pathologies.

The aim of this study was to investigate the epidemiological, clinical and therapeutic aspects of thoracic and vascular pathologies in the Andre FESTOC centre at the CHU-ME le Luxembourg in Bamako.

To achieve this goal we have set ourselves the following objectives:

II- Objectives

II.1- General objective :

- To study the ëpidëmio-clinical and therapeutic aspects of thoracic and vascular pathologies at the Andre FESTOC centre at the CHU-ME in Bamako.

II.2- Specific objectives :

- To determine the frequency of thoracic and vascular pathologies.
- Dë describe the management of thoracic and vascular pathologies.
- Analysing the results of thoracic and vascular pathology management.

III- Generalities :

III.1- Historical background:

III.1.1- History of surgery [11,12]

Term borrowed from ancient Greek is in the proper sense of the word one who does manual work "The surgeon". In other words, it was originally used to describe a doctor who heals with his hands as well as a e^шёте or a zither player.

This general and vague meaning was gradually lost. Already in the works of Hippocrates, but especially in the compilation of the Latin author Celsus, which date from around the Christian Гёre, we see that the term surgeon is used to designate a precise fagon of the physician who treated certain lesions by manual act (suturing wounds, reducing dislocations and fractures, dressing ulcers).

Prehistoric surgical practices even existed among primitive people. The study of excavations carried out in Lozère by Dr Prunier in 1873 revealed surgical practices on prehistoric skulls in the form of trepanation. These practices were more surgical than intentional, and existed in Egypt, Chaldean and China.

With Гёre of **Hippocrates** surgical practice really began in the 5th and **6th** century **BC**: fractured joints, mochlique, hemorrhoidal wound, fistula, where we see appear for the first time a treatise reporting surgical practice: reduction of a dislocation, reduction and contention of fractures, treatment of wounds.

Celsus wrote in the 3rd^e century BC that Herophitlie and Erasistratus carried out the first systematic human dissections, the basis of all serious anatomy But surgeons also carried them out. Certain operations such as autoplasties, penetrating abdominal wounds, operative cures of hydrocèles and hernias, and bladder pruning.

From the Christian Гёre (**131 -201 AD**) **Galen** made a correct description of the skeleton, joints and muscles of the limbs, but that of the vessels, nerves and viscères was mediocre instead.

In the **seventeenth** century we witness the creation of human anatomy as a true science. **Vesalius** denounced errors, successfully operated on purulent pleurisy and was one of the first to diagnose aortic aneurysm.

The discovery of the anaesthetic properties of lather and chloroform **in 1847**, and Lister's creation of the antiseptic method, profoundly transformed surgery. Guillaume **Dupytren** (**1777-1835**), a pupil of **Bichat**, is considered to be the creator of modern surgery. He resected the first lower jaw in **1812**, performed a subcutaneous tenotomy of the sterno-cleido-mastoi'dian for torticollis in **1812**, successfully performed iliac vascular ligations in **1815**, invented the enterostomy^, and became the first surgeon to perform a surgical operation on the lower jaw.

A few years earlier, in **1867**, Lister published statistics on his amputations with antisepsis.

Between **1870 and 1875**, surgical operations benefited from two major technical changes: general anaesthesia and, above all, the Listerian antiseptic method. This is referred to as the "true surgical revolution".

However, the creation of modern surgery was essentially a collective effort, thanks to publications and periodic international congresses, the first of which was held in Paris in 1867.

In 1886 **Chamberland** and then **Villard**, students of **Pasteur**, introduced the autoclave and the flaming oven, later modified by **Poupinel**;

In **1900, Champut** created sterilisable gloves. We are therefore witnessing an evolution from antisepsis to asepsis.

It is clear that in each country there have been more or less numerous and rapid individual developments.

We can now classify under three main headings the very large number of observations that will appear in great numbers and multiply rapidly over the next twenty-five or thirty years.

Operations that have existed for centuries and have never ceased to be performed, such as vascular ligations, superficial amputations, breast amputations, strangulated hernia operations, bladder pruning, cranial trepanations, emphysema operations, etc., are still performed today.

Operations that had previously been performed on an exceptional basis but were abandoned as too serious. These include hernia operation, nephrectomy and splenectomy,

1 amputation of the cervix and reparative vaginal surgery, abdominal surgery for ovarian cysts or even uterine fibroids.

Absolutely new operations that are increasing all the time. These included bone and joint surgery, which had remained just mutilating, and ostëotomies. Visceral surgery was created in just a few years with **Pean** in **1879** and **Bilroth** in **1880**.

This creative period also saw the emergence of specialities, thanks to the considerable improvements that were gradually made with the use of endoscopy and **X-rays** (Roentgen **1894**).

As a result, many entirely new instruments and devices were created from scratch, and operating techniques were developed and perfected.

III.1.2-   Developments in thoracic and vascular surgery :

Surgical practices on the vessels and thorax had existed for siëcles. In this section we will attempt to show revolution and the individualisation of thoracic and vascular surgery as a surgical speciality.

During the Christian era in the first century, **Gallien** performed vascular ligatures and cauterisation on vessels **[13]**. In **1546, Ambroise Pare** described vascular ligation techniques on bullet wounds.

Alexis Carrel described the triangulation suture in 1902. During the First World War, **Rene Leriche** performed arterial repairs **[13]**.

Sicard and **Forestier** developed the angiography technique for the first time in 1923 **[14]**.

In 1852, **Bowditch** reported the first successful thoracocentesis **by Wyman**.

During the First World War in **1918, Graham** and **Bell** achieved the first successful drainage of a pyothorax **[15]**.

With the development of the first prototype ventilator by **Brunnel** around the 1930s, certain procedures became possible. The first real pneumonectomy was performed by **Nissan, Hight** and **Graham** in **1932-1933 [15]**.

Techniques were improved and developed (dissection, ligation or suture of hilar structures) and there was a wide range of interventions. **Blalock** and **Ravitch** were the first to successfully drain the heart, while **Klassen** repaired a ruptured thoracic aorta **[15]**.

From then on, this speciality would see the development of new operative techniques and procedures, especially with the discovery of extracorporeal circulation by **Gibbon** in 1954 **[15]**.

Since 1960, a great deal of work has gone into revolutionising thoracic and vascular surgery.

The development of tracheal resection techniques by **Pearson** and **Grillo** in **1970** [15,16], the development of lung surgery techniques, and the introduction of thoracoscopy by **Miller** and **Daniel [15]**.
Skinne, **Belsey** and **Orringer** made contributions on surgery for resophageal pathology [17].

III.2- Reminders:

III.2.1-   Overview of the anatomy and function of the thorax [18] :
General topography of the thorax (walls and contents)
III.2.1.1-   The walls :
The walls of the thorax are ostëo-chondro-muscular
The skeleton is ostëo-cartilaginous (thoracic case).

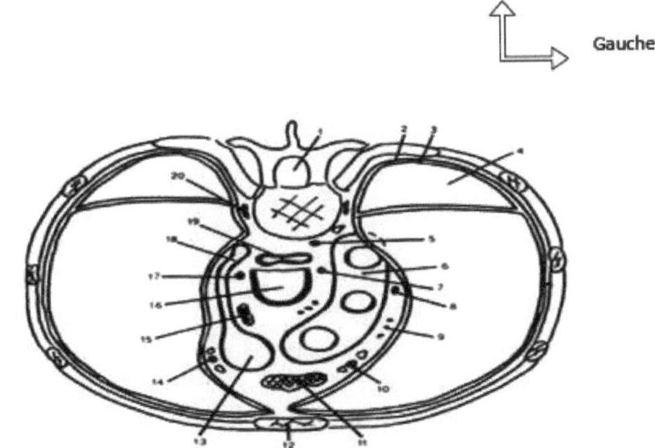

Figure 1 : Coupe horizontale du thorax en T4

1. 4ᵉ vertèbre thoracique (T4).
2. Plèvre pariétale.
3. Plèvre viscérale.
4. Poumon gauche.
5. Canal thoracique.
6. Crosse de l'aorte.
7. Nerf laryngé récurrent* gauche.
8. Nerf vague* gauche.
9. Plexus cardiaque superficiel.
10. Nerf phrénique gauche (et vaisseaux phréniques supérieurs*).
11. Thymus.
12. Sternum.
13. Veine cave supérieure.
14. Nerf phrénique droit.
15. Nœud lymphatique* de la crosse de la veine azygos*.
16. Trachée.
17. Nerf vague* droit.
18. Crosse de la veine azygos*.
19. Œsophage.
20. Sympathique thoracique.

Figure 1: Horizontal section of the thorax at T4

3.2.1.2- Constitution :

1. Behind (and on the median line): the vertebral column (1).
2. forward: the sternum (2).
3. laterally: the costal arches, i.e. 12 pairs of ribs (3) extended forward by the

3.2.1.4-   The anterior mediastinum.
Situated in front of the plane passing through the anterior face of the slice, this is the largest mediastinal sector, with 2 levels: lower (cardiac) and upper (supra-cardiac).

- The trachea (1) ;
- Le creur (2) ;
- Superior vena cava (3) ;
- Aortic arch (4) ;
- And bifurcation of the pulmonary artery (5) ;

- Brachiocephalic venous trunk (6) ;
- Arterial brachiocephalic trunk (7) ;
- The thymus (8) ;
- Phrenic nerves, right (9) and left (10).

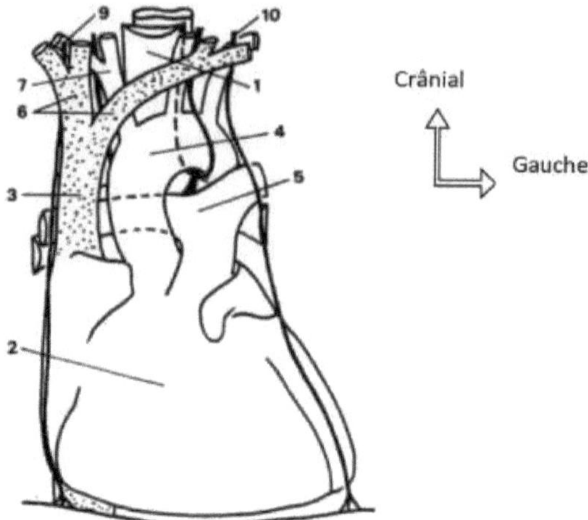

Figure 2: Anterior view of the mediastinum.

3.2.1.5-   The middle mediastinum.

Located between the 2 planes passing through the anterior and posterior faces of the trachea, it is a narrow, flattened, vertically elongated sector comprising 2 stages:
Superior, tracheobronchial and inferior: triangular ligaments of the lungs.
The trachea (1) ;
Triangular ligaments (2) ;
Main bronchi and pulmonary pëdiculi (3);
The aortic arch (4),
The left common carotid artery (5)
Branch of the azygos vein (6) ;
Left supëterior inter-costal vein (7);
The 2 vagus nerves (8, 9)

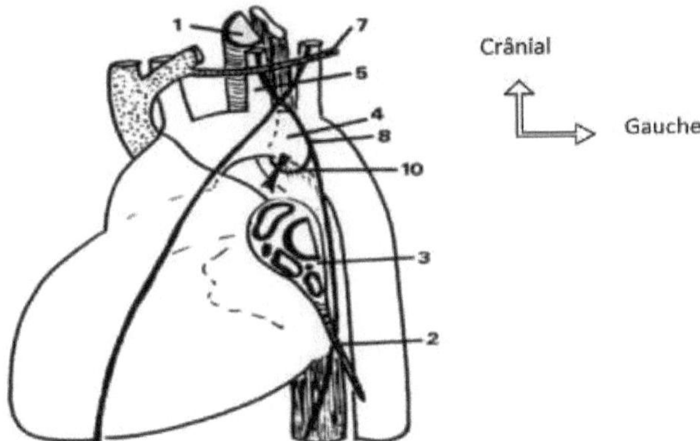

Figure 3: Left lateral view of the mediastinum.

3.2.1.6- **the thoracic cavity represents the osteo-cartilaginous skeleton limiting the cavity**
thoracic. It is made up of (Fig. 1, 2) :
- The sternum (1), in front ;
- The spinal column (2), in arridre ;
- The costal arches, ribs (3) and cartilage (4) laterally.

These pieces of bone are held together by :
- Joints;
- And muscles, in particular the intercostal muscles, which laterally join the ribs and costal cartilages (together forming the rib cage).

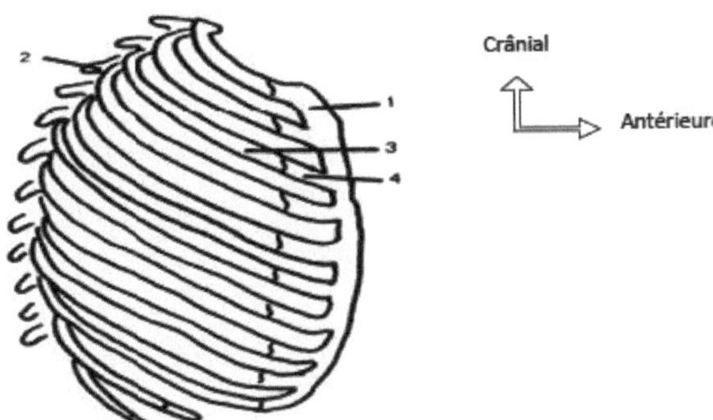

Figure 4 : Thoracic cage (side view). General configuration.

The thorax has the shape of a truncated cone, with a lower base, slightly flattened in the anterior-posterior direction, becoming roughly cylindrical in its lower part. In fact, the configuration varies according to the subject: narrow, in the long-bodied, or on the contrary wide in the short-bodied.

The rib cage can be described as follows:
- 4 sides,
- An upper orifice, or apex,
- A lower orifice, or base.

3.2.1.7-   **The upper thoracic opening.**

Limits.

Anteriorly, the jugular incision of the sternum (1), surmounted by the interclavicular ligament, and articulated laterally with the sternal extremity of the clavicle.

Behind, the upper edge of the first thoracic vertebra (2).

Laterally: the first dimension (3).

3.2.1.8-   **The lower thoracic opening :**

Limits :

1.   Ahead, the xiphoi'de process (1).
2.   Back: the 12eme thoracic vertebra (2).
3.   Laterally: the inferior chondrocostal rim (3); from back to front: the floating ribs, then the 10eme , 9eme , 8eme , 7eme costal cartilages.

3.2.1.11- Diaphragm :

The diaphragm is a niusculo-aponevTotic partition dividing the trunk into 2 ëtages (thorax above, abdomen below).

The diaphragm is a broad arch, looking down and forward, with an anterior portion (1), mobile, sternocostal, almost horizontal, ëvasëe in domes, on either side of the median line :

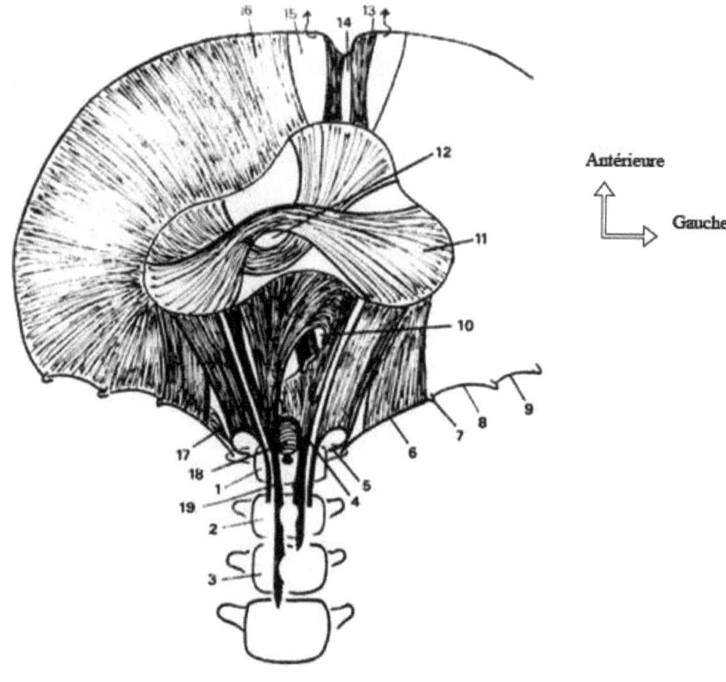

1. 1re vertèbre lombaire
2. 2e vertèbre lombaire.
3. 3e vertèbre lombaire
4. Pilier gauche.
5. Ligament arqué médial*.
6. Ligament arqué latéral*.
7. 12e côte.
8.9. Arcades intercostales (Senac)*.
10. Hiatus œsophagien
11. Centre tendineux.
12. Orifice de la V.C.I.
13. Partie sternale.
14. Fente rétroxiphoïdienne.
15. Fente de Larrey.
16. Partie costale.
17. Faisceau costoïdal.
18. Hiatus aortique.
19. Pilier droit.

Figure 5: Overall view of the diaphragm (lower face assumed to be reclined).

Vascularisation and innervation of the diaphragm :

Arteres :

I . the extreme functional importance of the diaphragm explains the richness of its vascularisation.

The top face of the diaphragm (1) receives :

- Branches of the musculo-phrenic artery (2), lateral terminal branch of the internal thoracic artery (3).
- The superior phrenic arteries (4) (derived from the internal thoracic arteries), satellites of the phrenic nerve (5).

Branches of the last 4 posterior intercostal arteries.

The underside (6) :

The inferior phrenic arteries (7), arising from the aorta above the diaphragm; ascending, they divide on the inferior surface of the centre of tendon into 3 branches (8) (anterior, middle and posterior), anastomosing into an arch from which branchlets graft to the centre of tendon arise.

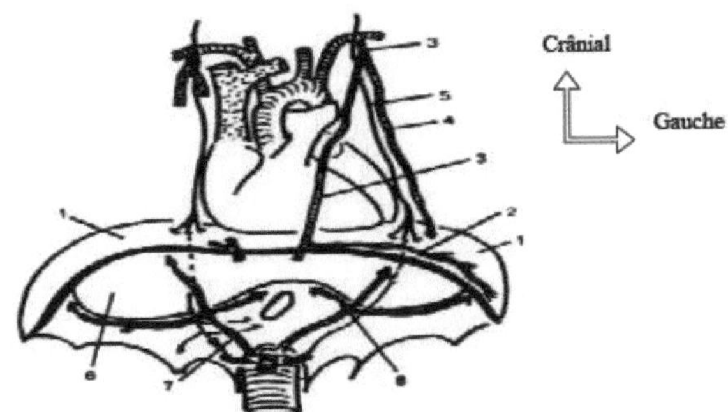

Figure 6: Arteries of the diaphragm (anterior view).

Veins :

- Whether or not they are satellites of the arteries, most of them drain into the phrenic veins, which are inferior and tributary to the IVC (just below the diaphragm).
- Certain venules join the resophageal veins or the veins of the liver ligaments (sickle or triangular), forming accessory portal veins.

Lymphatic :

There are 2 original networks:

1. the subpleural network (A) (from the upper surface) draining lymph towards the lymph nodes:

- Sternal (1), middle mëdiastinal (2), and postëterior (3),
- But also lumbar (4).

2.the sub-peritoneal network (B) (from the underside) draining the lymph to the lymph nodes:
- Phrenic infèrieurs, and lumbar (4);

But also sternal (retro-xiphoid) (trans-diaphragmatic collectors).
- We must therefore stress the importance of abdomino-thoracic lymphatic connections, which explain the trans-diaphragmatic spread of neoplastic or infectious processes.

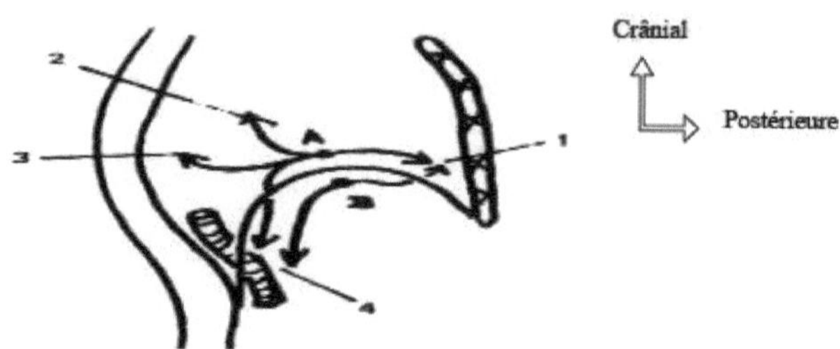

Figure 7: Lymphatic drainage (sagittal section).

Nerves :

1. the phrenic nerves (2 and 7) are the only motor nerves (each phrenic nerve innervates a hemi-diaphragm).

Upper diaphragm (1) ;

The right phrenic nerve (2) divides 3 cm outside the median line into 3 branches;

Front (3) ;

Lateral (4);

Posterieur (5);

Ganglions (Luska) (6);

The left phrenic nerve (7) ;

The other afferences are very incidental:

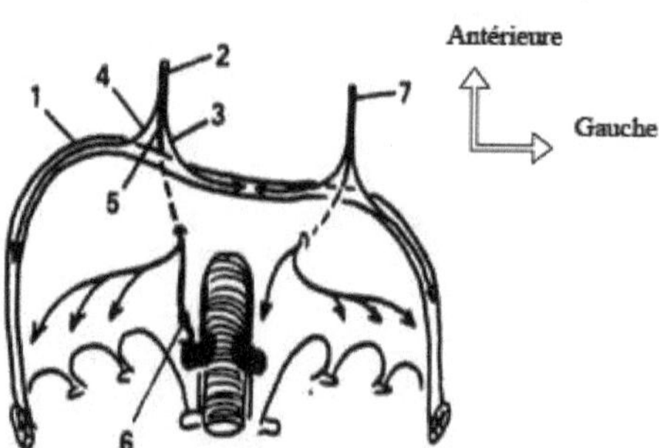

Figure 8: Terminal branches of the phrenic nerve (schematic anterior view).

3.2.2- Anatomical and functional overview of the circulatory system [19] :

Cardiovascular system :

The cardiovascular system is Гormё by the creur, which pulses blood through the body, and the blood vessels, which form a tight network of tubes carrying blood. There are three types of vessel:
- The arteries, which carry blood from the heart ;
- The veins, which carry the blood to the heart;

14

- The capillaries, which connect the arteries and veins, are the smallest of the blood vessels, and are where oxygen, nutrients and metabolic waste are exchanged with the tissues.

The walls of the blood vessels of the cardiovascular system are made up of three tunics:

- The tunica externa (adventitia) - the outer layer of connective tissue :
- The tunica media - the layer of smooth muscle (which may also contain variable clusters of elastic fibres in large and medium-sized arteries);
- The tunica interna (intima) - the internal endothelial layer in blood vessels.

Arteries themselves are subdivided into three classes, depending on the amount of smooth muscle and ëlastic fibres that contribute to the overall size of the vessel and its function.

- The large ëlastic arteries contain substantial quantities of ëlastic fibres in the media, which allow dilation and return to normal calibre during the cardiac cycle. This is involved in maintaining blood flow during diastole, 1 aorta, the brachiocephalic troc, the left common carotid artery, the left subclavian artery and the pulmonary artery trunk are examples.
- The middle muscular arteries are made up of a media containing a large number of smooth muscle fibres. This feature allows these vessels to regulate their diameter and control the flow of blood to different parts of the body. Examples of medium-sized muscular arteries are most of the truncular arteries, such as the femoral, axillary and radial arteries.
- The small arteries and arterioles control the filling of capillaries and contribute directly to blood pressure in the vascular system.

Veins are also subdivided into three classes:

Large veins contain smooth muscle fibres in the media. The superior vena cava, inferior vena cava and protective vein are examples.

- Small and medium veins contain small amounts of smooth muscle fibres, and the outer tunica is the thinnest. Examples of small and medium veins are the superficial veins of the upper and lower limbs, and the deep veins of the leg and forearm.
- Venules are the smallest veins and drain capillaries.

Although veins are similar to arteries in their general structure, there are a number of distinctive features.

- The walls of the veins, and more specifically the media, are thin.
- The endoluminal diameters of the veins are large.
- There are often several veins (comitant or satellite veins) in contact with the arteries in the peripheral regions. Valves are often present in the veins, particularly in the peripheral veins below the level of the hollow. These are often pairs of cusps that facilitate venous return to the crevice.

Lymphatic system :

Lymphatic vessels :

Lymphatic vessels form a complex and extensive network of interconnected channels, which begin as porous, blind lymphatic capillaries within the body's tissues, then converge to form several larger vessels that finally drain into large veins at the base of the neck.

The lymphatic vessels mainly collect the fluids lost by the capillary beds during nutrient exchange processes, and return them to the venous vascular system. Pathogens, lymphatic system cells, cellular products and debris are also contained in the interstitial fluid that drains into the lymphatic capillaries.

In the graft intestine, certain fats absorbed by the intestinal epithelium are incorporated into lipoprotein complexes (chylomicrons), which are released by the epithelial cells into the interstitial compartment. Along with other components of the interstitial fluid, the chylomicrons drain into the lymphatic capillaries (designed as lacteal capillaries in the grafted intestine) and are finally released into the venous system of the neck. The lymphatic system is therefore the main transport route for seeds absorbed by the intestine.

The fluid in most lymphatic vessels is clear and colourless, and is referred to as lymph. The fluid in the lymphatic vessels of the grafted intestine is lactescent due to the presence of chylomicrons; it is called chylous fluid.

Lymphatic vessels exist in most parts of the body, except in the brain, bone marrow and avascular tissues such as epithelium and cartilage.

Lymph movement in lymphatic vessels is mainly generated by the indirect action of adjacent structures, notably skeletal muscle contraction and arterial pulsations. Unidirectional flow is maintained by the presence of valves in the vessels.

Lymphatic nreiids :

Lymph nodes are small encapsulated structures (0.5 - 2.5 cm long) which interrupt the course of the lymphatic vessels and contain elements of the immune system, such as lymphocyte lines or macrophages. They act as elaborate filters that trap and phagocytose certain substances in the lymph. They also detect and defend against foreign antigens, which are also transported by the lymph.

Because lymph nodes ëare efficient filters and the flow through them ëis slow, cells that metastasise (migrate at a distance) from primary tumours and penetrate lymphatic vessels can lodge in lymph nodes and grow there as secondary tumours. Lymph nodes draining an area of infection or other pathology may enlarge and change, sometimes becoming 'hard' or 'tender'. These changes can help clinicians detect pathology or look for spread of disease.

A number of areas of the body have a large number of lymph nodes. Naturally, the nodes in most of these areas drain the body's surface, the digestive system and the respiratory system. These three regions are high-risk sites for the penetration of foreign pathogens.

Lymph nodes are numerous and can be palpated in the axilla, groin and femoral regions, as well as in the neck. Deep sites, which are not palpable, include nodes associated with the trachea and bronchi in the thorax, and the aorta and its branches in the abdomen.

Trunks and lymphatic channels :

All the lymphatic vessels converge to form larger trunks or channels, which drain into the venous system in the neck, where the internal jugular veins join the subclavian veins to form the brachiocephalic veins.

• Lymph from the right side of the head and neck, the right upper limb, the right side of the thorax and the right side of the upper and superficial regions of the abdominal wall is carried by the lymphatic vessels which drain into the veins of the right side of the neck;

• Lymph from other parts of the body is carried by the lymphatic vessels, which drain into the veins on the left side of the neck.

4- Signs of the pathologies studied :

4.1- Thoracic pathologies :

4.1.1- Pleural effusions [20] :

4.1.1.1- Definition :

Pleural effusion is the abnormal accumulation of fluid or gas in the pleural space (the area between the two layers of the thin membrane covering the lungs).

4.1.1.2-   Etiologies :

Many conditions can lead to pleural ëpurgation. Some of the common causes (ranked from most common to least common) include

• Heart failure, tumours, pneumonia, pulmonary embolism, surgery such as recent coronary artery bypass grafting, chest trauma, cirrhosis, renal failure, systëmic lupus ërythëmateux, pancreatitis, rheumatoid arthritis, tuberculosis, nephrotic syndrome, përitonëal dialysis.

• Drugs such as: hydralazine, procainamide, isoniazid, phenytoin, chlorpromazine, methysergide, interleukin-2, nitrofurantoin, bromocriptine, dantrolene and procarbazine.

4.1.1.3-   Symptoms :

Many people with pleural effusion are completely asymptomatic. The most frequent symptoms, whatever the type of effusion in the pleural cavity or the cause, are :

• Shortness of breath

• Chest pain

Paraclinical examination

• Chest X-ray and/or ultrasound scan

• Laboratory analyses carried out on a liquid sample

Depending on the cause, the liquid may be either :

• Rich in protein (exudate)

• Aqueous (transudate)

• Sometimes CT angiography.

4.1.2- Pericarditis [21] :

The pericardium is a fibrous sac containing the heart muscle and the roots of the large blood vessels. When the heart muscle contracts, part of the pericardium secretes a liquid (varying in quantity from 30 to 50 ml), which acts as a lubricant. In the event of inflammation of the pericardium, this fluid can increase and prevent the heart muscle from contracting; this is known as pericarditis.

A distinction must be made between acute and chronic përicarditis. The former is an inflammation that occurs following a viral infection and gënëralisëe. Then, chronic përicarditis occurs when one or more inflammations of the përicard occur following the first.

4.1.2.1-   Symptoms

Most symptoms are not specific. There are, however, some that are common, depending on whether the condition is chronic or chronic.

The symptoms are the same as those following a viral infection:

• Fever, muscle and joint pain, sweating

• Pain in the thorax, accompanied by radiation into the ëpaules and jaw

• Palpitations and increased heart rate

• Dyspnoea (difficulty breathing), dizziness, even loss of consciousness following a slowing of the heartbeat, or even complete cessation of the heartbeat.

4.1.2.2-   Causes:

• Pathogenic agents such as viruses or bacteria

• Cancers (especially of the lungs, mammary gland and lip)

• Infections of all kinds, such as tuberculosis.

In most cases, no cause is found for the inflammation, which is referred to as idiopathic pericarditis.

4.1.2.3-   - Diagnosis :

After an interview with the patient, during which he or she is familiarised with his or her medical history and symptoms, the cardiologist carries out a number of clinical examinations and looks for any signs of pericarditis or complications.

•   Electrocardiogram :

It records the electrical activity of the heart using different electrodes placed on the hands, feet and chest.

•   Cardiac ultrasound :

This examination is carried out quickly in the patient's bed. It easily detects any increase in the volume of fluid around the creura and measures the impact of the fluid on the work of the creura.

•   Scanner and magnetic resonance imaging (MRI)

They allow us to observe the thickening of the pericardium, but also the gene of the work of the ventricles in the case of constrictive pericarditis.

4.1.3- Firm trauma to the thorax [22] :

Thoracic trauma is damage to the chest wall and the organs inside the rib cage as a result of impact, accident or exertion. They may be penetrating (open) or internal (closed) and cause injury to several organs: the heart, large vessels, lung, resophagus, trachea, etc. In the case of thoracic trauma, priority is given to treating those parts of the body affected that are life-threatening.

Simple rib fracture is the most common thoracic trauma. A chest X-ray can detect any associated lesions, such as pneumothorax. The treatment of a fractured rib is not always surgical. In the case of simple fractures, painkillers are prescribed and the bone heals itself in the following weeks.

4.1.4- Endothoracic goitre [22] :

Goitre is a condition of the thyroid gland, characterised by an increase in size of the thyroid gland, slightly below the Adam's apple. Sometimes a family affliction, it affects women more than men and increases in frequency with age. Inhabitants of mountainous regions are more affected because of a deficiency of iodine in the soil (an essential element in thyroid hormones). In Switzerland, as in other developed countries, iodine-enriched dietary salt has helped to reduce the number of goitres. It should be noted that congenital factors or certain conditions can also cause goitres.

Apart from their unaesthetic appearance, most goitres are benign and do not generally interfere with the normal function of the thyroid gland. However, enlargement of this gland can lead to compression of neighbouring organs and impair swallowing (dysphagia), speech (dysphonia) or breathing (dyspnea).

Treatment varies according to the cause and severity of the goitre. The goitre may remain small, without influencing hormone secretion or creating compression. In this case, regular endocrinological monitoring is suggested, including palpation, ultrasound and blood tests. Surgical treatment is indicated in the case of very unpleasant or bothersome goitres in the neck, leading to hyperthyroidism. The operation involves complete or partial removal of the gland (thyroidectomy).

4.1.5- Diaphragmatic hernia [22] :

Diaphragmatic hernias are protrusions of abdominal contents into the thorax through a hole in the diaphragmatic cupola. Compression of the lungs can lead to persistent pulmonary hypertension. Diagnosis is based on the thorax.

4.2- Vascular pathologies :

4.2.1- Arteriopathies :

4.2.1.1- **Definition** [13] :

I . arteritis is an inflammatory lesion of an artery, but inflammatory arteritis is any lesion of an artery.

4.2.1.2- **Etiologies and risk factors** [23] :

Arteriopathy can have different causes.

- Degenerative arteriopathies are linked to atherosclerosis due to excess cholesterol;
- Acute arterial ischemia is generally due to thrombosis (blood clot);
- Arterial aneurysm ;
- Other forms: inflammatory diseases (Horton's disease, Takayasu's disease, Buerger's disease, trauma, compressions, infectious diseases, etc).

4.2.1.3- **Symptoms**

4.2.1.3.1- Atheromatous plaque can cause arterial dilatation or stenotic lesions. A stenosis may be manifested by an increase in circulatory velocity and a decrease in pressure downstream of the stenosis during effort, with increased flow.

4.2.1.3.2- **Arteriopathies of the upper limbs** [24]

Compared with arteriopathies of the lower limb, arteriopathies of the upper limb are rare. They often occur in Horton's disease.

4.2.1.3.3- **Symptoms**

They are often asymptomatic, but may manifest as Raynaud's syndrome or painful permanent digital ischaemia, more rarely as claudication of the MS or hand (sometimes, rarely typical). Acute forms are manifested by :

- Acute arterial obliteration with or without sensory-motor ischemia;
- Acute ischaemic syndrome (pain, coldness, warmth and acral paresis).

4.2.1.4- **Paraclinical examinations** :

4.2.1.4.1- **Doppler ultrasonography**: a non-invasive examination that provides a morphological and hemodynamic study of the arterial network. It is the first additional examination requested by the practitioner in the event of obliterative arteriopathy of the lower limbs. It is the examination of choice for monitoring revascularisation (endovascular or surgical) or for detecting asymptomatic lesions in certain categories of patient (diabetic patients in particular).

4.2.1.4.2- **Angioscanner**: increasingly used by vascular surgeons, gives excellent information on the arterial tree from the aorta to the proximal thirds of the leg arteries. It requires the injection of iodine. It enables the arterial wall to be studied and calcifications to be visualised; these calcifications can lead to interpretation being affected by the "blooming effect".

4.2.1.4.3- **Magnetic Resonance Angiography (MRA)**: highly effective for visualising the arteries of the lower limbs. This examination does not require the injection of iodine and there is no artefact with calcium, so it is particularly suitable for diabetic or renal failure patients with distal arterial lesions.

4.2.1.4.4- **Arteriography**: invasive and increasingly impractical. The vascular surgeon requests this examination if the information obtained from magnetic resonance angiography or angioscanner is not sufficient. It is usually carried out in the operating theatre or procedure room at the same time as the therapeutic procedure. Arteriography provides very precise mapping of arterial lesions.

4.2.2- Arteriovenous fistulas :

4.2.2.1-   Definition [25] :

The **arteriovenous fistula** (AVF) is a **vascular approach** used primarily in the treatment of renal failure and hemodialysis.

4.2.2.2-   Paraclinical examination [26] :

Echodoppler is the paraclinical examination of choice, enabling the majority of creation and dysfunction problems to be resolved. The three-part echodoppler assessment - arterial, venous and soft tissue surrounding this network - enables the best site of creation to be chosen and certain evolving problems to be anticipated. From the moment the arteriovenous fistula (AVF) is created, clinical monitoring and echodoppler - the only non-invasive method providing flow measurement - should detect complications and assess maturation before the first puncture or the need for any superficialisation. When development is apparently clinically inadequate, with an arterialised vein that is barely visible or palpable, or with thrill abnormalities, ultrasound can be used to distinguish between a true delay and a pseudo-delay in maturation, due to excessive soft tissue thickness that is accessible to superficialisation or ultrasound-guided puncture. The main aim of monitoring is to prevent loss of vascular access due to thrombosis, which in most cases is caused by stenosis. Calculation of flow rate (Q), an essential part of the assessment of an AVF using echodoppler, can relate an isolated drop in flow rate to a possible stenosis or rule it out. Hyperflow, which begins above 1500 ml/min, is all too often overlooked, despite the fact that it can lead to cardiac decompensation, pulmonary hypertension, ischaemia or aneurysmal degeneration. Associated with intermediate or proximal stenosis, it generates or increases venous hyperpressure. Distal ischaemia, suspected on the basis of clinical data, is assessed using echodoppler, supplemented by digital pressure readings, which enable a positive diagnosis to be made (< 60 mmHg and finger-arm index < 0.4). Problems arising during dialysis sessions - difficult cannulation, aspiration of blood clots, insufficient flow, local pain, prolonged bleeding - raise the suspicion of stenosis: these can be observed outside the clinic in more than a third of cases, where ultrasound avoids unnecessary fistulography.

4.2.3- Deep vein thrombosis [27] :

4.2.3.1-   Definition :

Deep vein thrombosis is the result of a blood clot forming in a large-diameter vein in the legs, arms, abdomen, etc. Deep vein thrombosis is a medical emergency because of its potentially serious complications.

4.2.3.2-   Etiology and risk factors :

All people who, for one reason or another, experience a significant reduction in their mobility are at risk of venous thrombosis: illnesses or accidents resulting in immobilisation or paralysis, the fitting of a cast, people confined to bed for several days without being able to get up, and so on.

In addition, certain categories of people have a higher risk of venous thrombosis:
- People aged over 75 ;
- People who have already had problems with thrombosis or varicose veins;
- People who suffer from obësité ;
- Women taking restrogënes (contraceptive pill or menopause treatment);

- People who have recently had a myocardial infarction or a (stroke or "cerebral attack", particularly if it causes partial paralysis);
- People who have undergone surgery, particularly orthopaedic surgery (e.g. hip or knee replacement);
- People suffering from cancer (five times higher risk);
- People suffering from severe cardiac or respiratory insufficiency ;
- Pregnant women, at the end of pregnancy and after giving birth (risk five to ten times higher);
- People who have a pacemaker or a central venous catheter (e.g. to administer chemotherapy);
- People suffering from a chronic inflammatory disease (lupus, Crohn's disease, etc.) or sepsis (generalized infection);
- People who smoke.

4.2.3.3- Symptoms :

A phlebitis close to the skin causes redness above the affected vein, which is warm, painful and sometimes swollen. On palpation, it feels like a hard cord where the vein is blocked. Phlebitis of a large vein causes **severe pain in the calf or thigh**, and sometimes the arm. Cramps, numbness or a sensation of heat in the affected limb may be felt. But in half the cases, deep vein thrombosis causes few symptoms, or even goes unnoticed.

In cases where the clot severely blocks blood circulation, the limb is swollen and the skin is taut, shiny and of a whitish or bluish hue. When deep vein thrombosis affects the calf, the person may feel a sharp pain when raising the toe towards the knee (known as the "Homans sign"). A mild fever (38°C) may also be present.

The appearance of these symptoms warrants an urgent medical consultation. Under no circumstances should the painful area be massaged, as this may dislodge the clot from the vein wall.

4.2.3.4- Paraclinical examinations :

4.2.3.4.1- Echodoppler or Doppler ultrasonography is an examination that examines veins and arteries and visualises a possible clot in a blood vessel. This examination uses ultrasound and takes between 15 and 30 minutes. It does not require local or general anaesthetic, or the injection of any products.

4.2.4- Venous insufficiency [28] :

4.2.4.1- Definition :

Venous insufficiency is due to poor circulation of blood to the heart.

4.2.4.2- Symptomatology :

Venous insufficiency is the cause of many symptoms, which intensify during the day and disappear after a night's lying down.

Venous insufficiency has various symptoms:

- Swelling, feeling of heaviness in the leg, tingling, itching, pain, night cramps, redness, feeling of impatience in the leg (irrepressible need to move the leg immediately).

The symptoms of venous insufficiency intensify during the day:

- They reach their peak intensity in the evening.
- Usually in the morning, after a night lying down, they have disappeared.
- They reappear gradually over the course of the day, depending on physical exertion.

4.2.4.3-   Paraclinical examination :

Venous echo-doppler: this is the gold standard test for diagnosing the quality and quantity of venous reflux and venous obliteration, and for determining its location (deep or superficial).

4.2.5- compartment syndrome [29] :

Compartmental syndrome is caused by an increase in pressure in an inextensible aponeurotic compartment, leading to muscular ischemia in the compartment. The first symptom is pain, regardless of the extent of the trauma. The diagnosis is clinical and is usually confirmed by measuring the pressure in the muscle compartment.

5- Treatment

Treatment of thoracic and vascular pathologies

5.1-   Purpose of treatment :

* Correcting anatomical dësorders
* Rëtablir correct hëmodynamics
* Improving symptoms
* Preventing and treating complications

5.2-   Treatment means and methods

5.2.1- Medical treatment

5.2.1.1-   Hygienic and dietetic measures

Rest adapted to the clinical stage, a low-salt diet (2 to 4 grams per 24 hours), a low-calorie diet in obese patients and the continuation of regular physical exercise unless contraindicated. And the prescription of parenteral or per-osteal molecules adapted to the pathology presented by the patient.

5.2.2- Surgical treatment

5.2.2.1-   Equipment

5.2.2.1.1-   Installation [30] :

Decubitus: patient lying down

* Dorsal: on the back ;
* Lateral: on the side ;
* Ventral: on the stomach.

-Proclive: the surface is inclined, head upwards.

-Trendelenburg: the surface is tilted head down.

Patients may also be in the sitting, standing, lithotomy or gynaecological position.

The operating tables can be articulated to allow angulation of the patient's body or part of the body.

5.2.2.1.2-   Approach

5.2.2.1.2.1- Thoracic surgery [31] :

5.2.2.1.2.1.1- Thoracotomy: Opening of the thorax through an intercostal space, the patient is in lateral dëcubitus more or less proпопcë depending on whether it is postëro-latëral or antero-lateral, the diseased lung becomes superior, the healthy lung inferior the inferior arm is placed in a padded trough, perpendicular to the operating table.

5.2.2.1.2.1.1.1-   Postero-lateral thoracotomy (PLT) and lateral thoracotomy (LT): This is the most commonly used approach. It most often passes through the 5th intercostal space, freeing the intercostal muscles and disengaging the 5th costal arch by displacing the scapula. Incision of the muscle groups: Trapeze- Latis dorsalis and Rhomboi'de- Latis dentele. For closure, muscle reconstitution, suture of the teguments and closure of the costal wall.

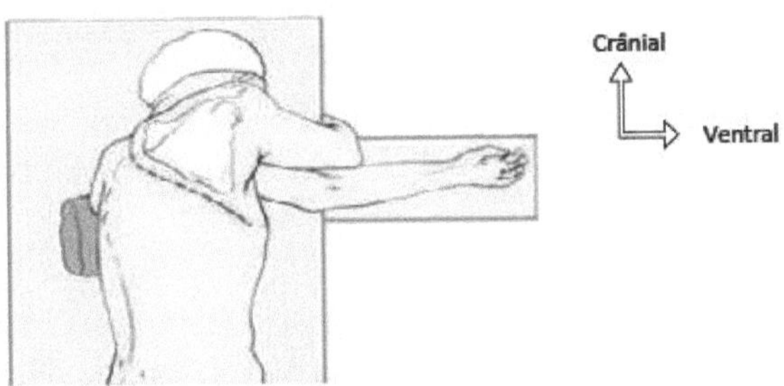

Figure 9: Posterolateral thoracotomy (PLT).

There are other ways and techniques of approaching the thorax:

- Clanchell and hemi-clanchell
- Anterior and antero-lateral thoracotomy;
- Bithoracotomy ;
- Direct thoracoscopy ;
- Surgical thoracoscopy video ;
- Video-assisted thoracic surgery (VAST) or video-assisted mini thoracotomy;
- Video assistance in conventional surgery;
- Robotics.

Direct thoracoscopy is based on the principles described by Jacobeus in 1910.

It uses a simple thoracoscope with a cold light that is inserted into the thorax using a trocar.

The surgeon has a direct view of the pleural cavity through the thoracoscope lens.

5.2.2.1.2.1.2- Thoracic drainage approach [30] :

5.2.2.1.2.1.2.1- The axillary route :

The puncture zone is dëlimitëe by the triangle of sëcuritë. This triangle is defined, in aтѐre by the postëterior axillary line, inferiorly by the level of the nipple (5th intercostal space) and anteriorly by the postëterior border of the pectoralis major. The point of insertion corresponds to the 4th intercostal space on the upper or middle axillary line. The main risk is of draining too low and leserating the diaphragmatic dome as well as the underlying intra-abdominal organs. The axillary route is theoretically the best way of draining a liquid pleural effusion.

5.2.2.1.2.1.2.2- The earlier route

It is located on the mid-clavicular line at the level of the 2nd intercostal space. If the drainage is too internal, there is a risk of damaging the internal mammary artery. It has the disadvantage of weighing down the pectoralis major muscle and the very unaesthetic nature of the scars generated. It is used in the drainage of a hëmothorax in the polytraumatisë patient and pneumothorax.

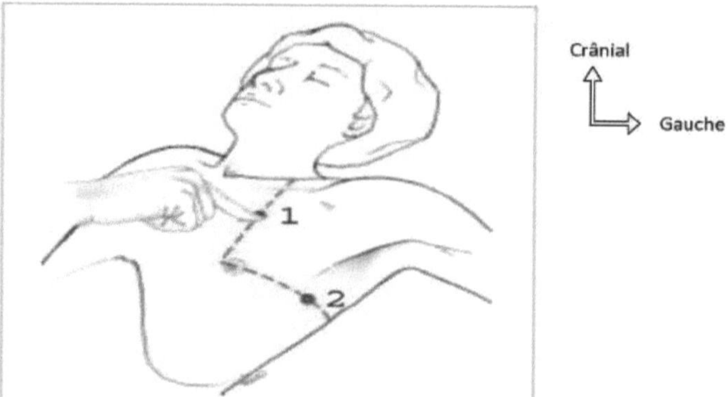

Figure 10: Thoracic drainage approaches (**1**. anterior approach, **2**. axillary approach). [32]

5.2.2.1.2.2- Vascular surgery

Brachial artery :

Approach at the elbow crease :

The distal part of the brachial artery and the origin of the radial and ulnar arteries can be approached. The arm is abducted at 90°, in external rotation, with the forearm extended and supinated. Passage of the elbow flexion fold requires a bayonet or elongated S-shaped incision. The superficial veins of the venous M should be preserved if possible, particularly when an approach for hëmodialysis is used. Once the superficial aponeurosis has been covered, the aponeurotic expansion of the biceps brachii muscle appears, stretched obliquely downwards and medially. A Ыдёге pronation allows this expansion to relax which facilitates its section. The brachial artery then appears, running between two white cords: medially the median nerve, laterally the pulse allows control of the brachial bifurcation, after reclining inferiorly and medially the round pronator muscle. The radial artery appears as an extension of the branchial artery and the first few centimetres of the ulnar artery are visible before it enters under the round pronator muscle and the epitrochlear muscles. There are very few sources of error in this approach. The only difficulty is appreciating the middle of the anterior aspect of the elbow. To do this, it is sufficient to correct the internal rotation of the arm and to avoid incising on the lateral edge of the biceps brachii muscle.

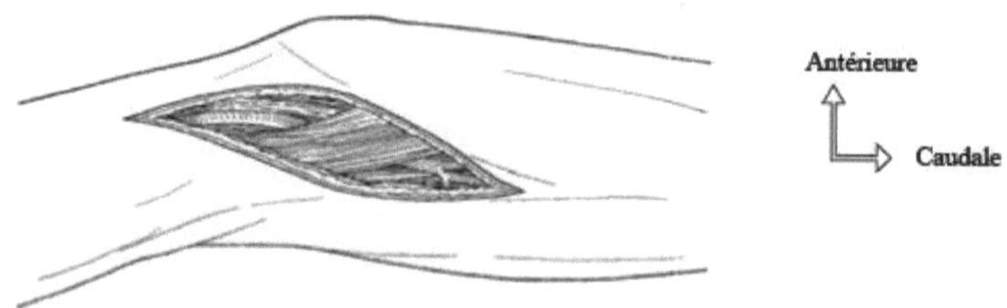

Figure 11: Approach to the brachial artery at the elbow. The aponeurotic exposure of the biceps brachii muscle pre-crosses the artery.

1.1.1.1.1.1.1.3- **THE RADIAL ARTERY (radialis)** [33]: first its external limit: tendons of the long abductor and the short extensor of the thumb. Then its internal limit: tendon of the long extensor of the thumb - at the palm of the hand: it crosses the upper end of the first intermetacarpal space and enters the interosseous compartment by inserting itself between the two fascicles of the adductor of the thumb. Vertical anti-brachial incision centred on the radial vein, after reclining the supinator longus. Approach of the radial artery between its two satellites.

1.1.1.1.1.1.1.4- SURGICAL APPROACH TO THE CUBITAL ARTERY [33] : Vertical extension of the approach to the humeral bifurcation, centred on the interosseous membrane.

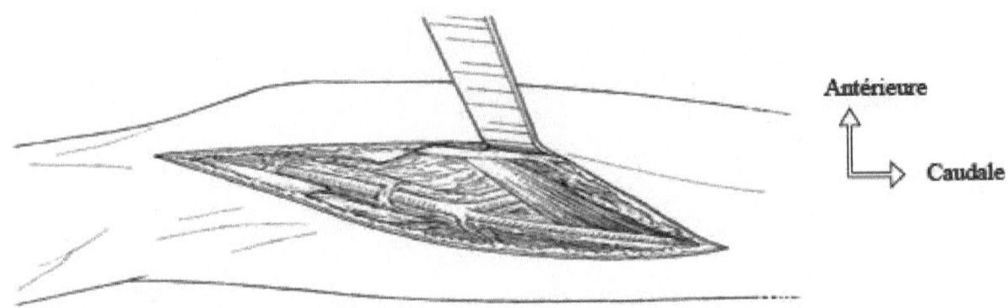

Figure 12: An aponeurotic expansion of the biceps transects the brachial artery over a few centimetres, extending the incision downwards to control the radial artery and the first few centimetres of the ulnar artery.

5.2.2.1.2.2.3- Abdominal aorta [34] :

Conventional approaches :

5.2.2.1.2.2.3.1-   Trans-peritoneal routes

Xipho-umbilical midline laparotomy

The operating field includes the entire abdomen and Scarpa's two triangles. A transverse block is placed under the point of the shoulder blades. The surgeon is positioned to the left of the patient, with the two assistants opposite. The cutaneous incision is a median xipho-subumbilical laparotomy, starting from the tip of the xiphoi'de apophysis, bypassing the umbilicus on the left, and stopping subumbilically at a variable distance from the pubic symphysis depending on the revascularisation procedure and the patient's morphology. Once the laparotomy has been performed, the retractors are inserted. For this approach, we use an auto-static retractor with removable valves of different depths. We also use two self-tracting valves that rest on the upper and lower edges of the laparotomy, thus improving and stabilising the upward and downward exposure. After fitting the retractors, the first step is to check that there are no visceral or hepatic lesions. The transverse colon and its mesocolon are folded upwards and covered with wet fields, and the grafted handles protected by a field are tilted to the right.

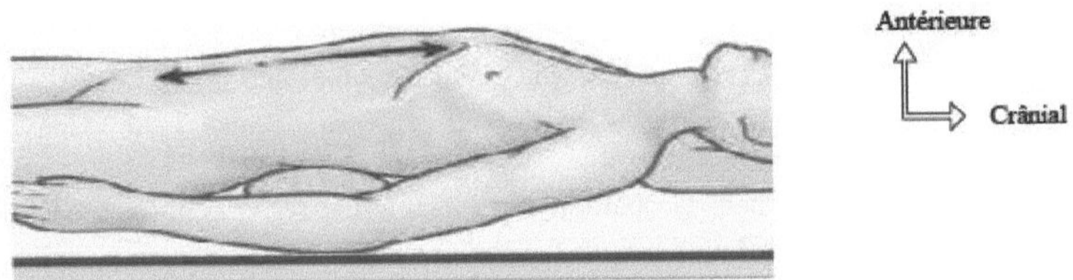

Figure 13: Median xiphopubic laparotomy approach. The patient is positioned with a transverse block placed at the base of the thorax.

5.2.2.1.2.2.3.1.1-   Exposure of the abdominal aorta

The aorta is approached by incising the pCTitoneum panëlal post^teriorly from bottom to top on the mëdian line while ascending towards the duodënojëjunal angle the tensioning of the first jёjunal loop facilitates section of the ligament of Treitz.

The duodёnum is l'ёcГтё on the right. Incision of the presacral lamina allows control of the aortic bifurcation. This incision is latёralisёe on the right in order to respect the pre sacral nerve plexus as much as possible.

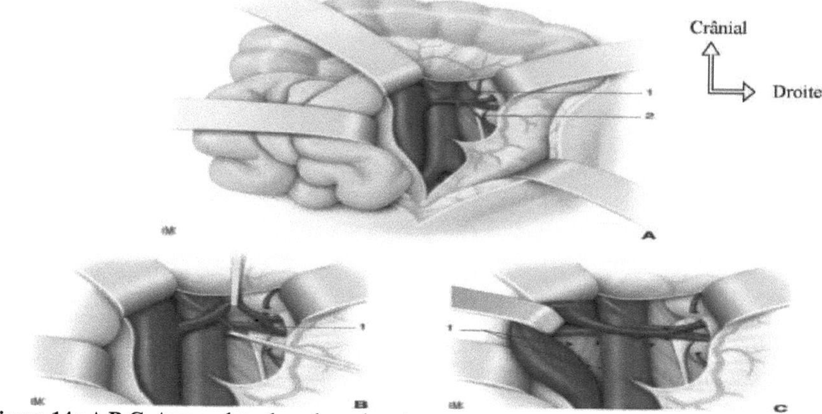

Figure 14 : A,B,C. Approach to the subrenal aorta.

5.2.2.1.2.2.4- Lower limb arteries [33] :

5.2.2.1.2.2.4.1- Femoral trigone approach:

Aseptic preparation of the entire lower limb has the advantage of allowing flexion or extension of the knee on demand. The operative field extends upwards over the pёri-umbilical region, incorporating the pelvis, the pubis and the controlatёral fёmoral axis. The surgeon is positioned on the side of the intestricate limb, with the assistant opposite. The instrument table is placed at the patient's feet. Exposure of the common fёmoral artery, the proximal superficial fёmoral artery, and the first segment of the deep fёmoral artery, allows excellent control of the fёmoral tripod. Our preference is for the mёdian incision bisecting the infёternal angle of the femoral trigone, situated midway between the anterior and suprailiac iliac crest and the pubic tubercle; it leads directly to the femoral vessels (). The cuUure incision is tegereously arciform and rises above the groin fold. The more or less thick subcutaneous cellular tissue comprises two layers: a superficial adipose layer and a deep layer rich in vascular elements (pudendal and circumflex arterial branches, greater saphenous vein and its associated branches). There are many superficial inguinal lymph nodes in this region, and hemostasis and lymphostasis performed with the electric scalpel and/or by ligatures must be rigorous. This is an essential part of the exposure: neglected, it can lead to excessively embarrassing post-operative lymphorrhea.

The vascular sheath is approached by opening and incising the femoral aponeurosis, leading directly to the vascular-nervous bundle, with the femoral nerve, femoral artery, femoral vein and deep lymph nodes, including Cloquet's lymph node, located at the innermost part of the crural ring. Arterial dissection is started close to the inguinal ligament and performed from top to bottom to facilitate control of the proximal segment of the deep femoral artery. The dangers of this approach are represented by the femoral nerve or its branches, and by venous elements that may be injured during control of the deep femoral artery.

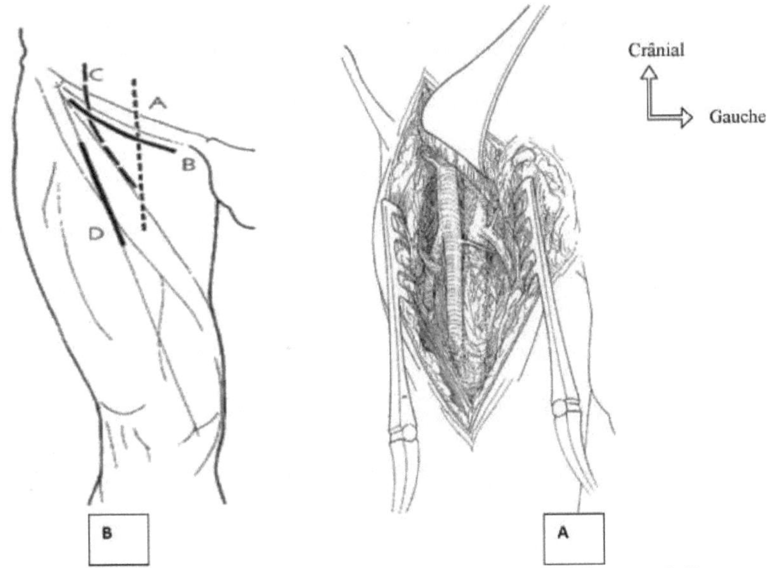

gure 15 : A. (A. median vertical approach, B. inguinal approach, C. external approach, D. antero-lateral approach).
B. Displacement of the celluloganglion during the vertical approach to the femoral tripod.

5.2.2.1.2.2.4.2-   Popliteal artery [33] :

Extended mediation:

The middle popliteal artery is rarely approached internally; the postëterior approach gives better daylight without muscle breakdown. Combined with the approaches to the upper and lower popliteal arteries, the medial approach to the middle popliteal artery allows an extended approach to the popliteal artery, at the cost of significant muscle sections. The cutaneous and subcutaneous incision combines the trace of the incisions of the high and low routes described above. The middle popliteal artery, which runs through the inter-condylar notch, is covered by the tendons of the muscles of the crow's feet, by the semimembranosus muscle, and then by the medial bundle of the gastrocnemius muscle, which inserts onto the medial femoral condyle. Traditionally, these muscles can be sectioned in their lower tendinous portion, and the ends marked on the wire can be repaired at the end of the operation. Five to six centimetres of the middle popliteal artery can be fully exposed. The collateral arteries must be respected. Branchereau proposes a technique for exposing the middle popliteal artery by isolating the muscles of the crow's feet and the semimembranosus muscle on lakes and cutting the reflex and recurrent fibres of the latter. The osteoperiosteal insertion block of the Sartorius, semitendinosus, gracilis and semimembranosus muscles is reinserted through the rugin to the tibial crete and sectioned. The medial bundle of the gastrocnemius muscle is either mobilised or sectioned to expose the middle popliteal artery. At the end of the operation, the osteoperiosteal block is reinserted with a Blount-type staple. The repair of these muscular tendons, whether severed or uninserted, warrants post-operative immobilisation of the knee in a flat splint.

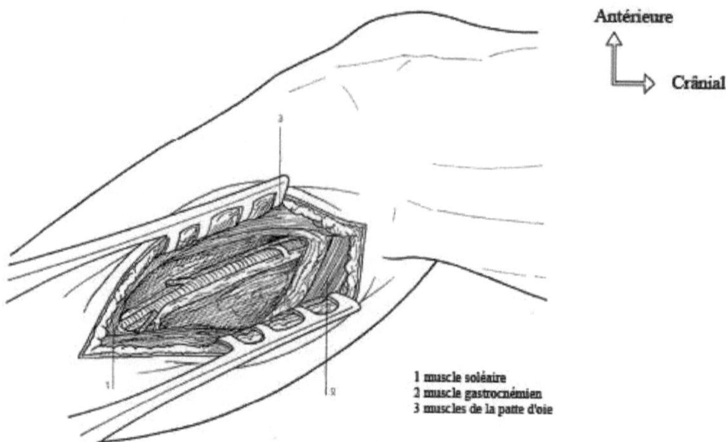

Figure 16. Exposure of the lower popliteal artery via the medial (or medial lateral) approach.

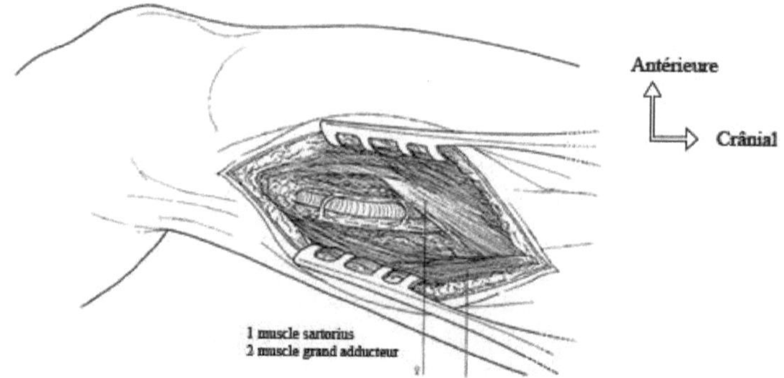

Figure 17: Medial (or medial lateral) approach to the upper popliteal artery Veins [33] :

5.2.2.1.2.2.4.3-   Long saphenous vein :

The patient is positioned supine, with the table leg raised 20 to 30 degrees. The lower limb rests on the buttock and the heel is slightly abducted and externally rotated. The operator is positioned medially and the assistant externally. The table is tilted 20 degrees towards the surgeon. The saphenofemoral junction is approached by a skin incision centred on a point two centimetres outside and below the pubic tubercle (). The incision is three to five centimetres long, and the external extremity lies just medial to the femoral artery, the pulse of which is located. The inguinal skin fold should not be cut, particularly in obese patients. We prefer to use a parallel incision above the fold, especially in women. The subcutaneous cellular tissue and superficial aponeurosis are incised along a transverse axis. The two retractors are then placed perpendicular to the axis of the incision. The VSI is located within the underlying adipose elements. It is easy to identify; it should not be found by transverse dissection in order to avoid lesioning the lymphatic elements, but by dissection distally in the axis of the limb. This involves dissection of the VFC on either side of the presumed saphenofemoral junction. In some cases, the superficial lateral pudendal artery may lie above the terminal portion of the saphenofemoral junction, making dissection difficult. In the event of difficulty, it may be necessary to section the artery; it is preferable to uncross it, particularly in men. The approach to the trunk of the VSI is extremely easy throughout its course. After incising the skin and subcutaneous cellular tissue, the VSI is easily identified. The approach is facilitated by per-operative ultrasound mapping, which is particularly recommended in adipose patients.

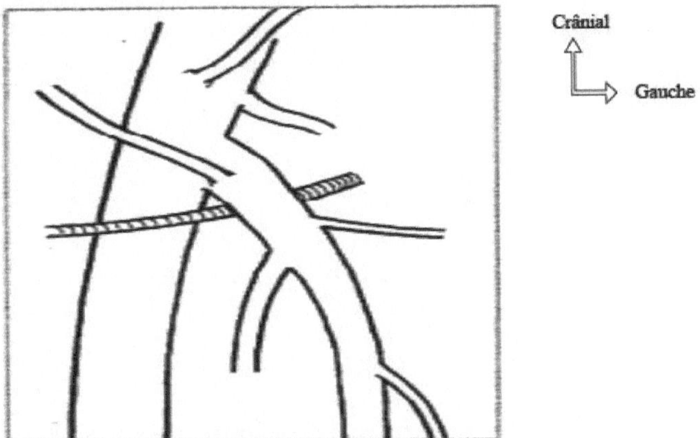

Figure 18: Saphenofemoral junction showing the arch of the VSI and its tributaries, noting the junction with the superficial lateral pudendal artery.

5.2.2.1.2.2.4.4-   Long saphenous vein [33] :

In the case of a unilateral approach, the surgeon is positioned in lateral decubitus, with the opéтe limb in the superior position and the table tilted 30 degrees towards the assistant. In case of bilateral approach the surgeon is installed in ventral decubitus. We feel that supine positioning of the surgeon is only justified when the same patient has both internal and external eveinage, or when the VSE terminates in the VSI or VFS without any connection with the popliteal fossa. To approach the termination of the VSE, the level of the skin incision is determined by the topography of the saphenopopliteal junction identified beforehand by echodoppler. The cutaneous incision is transverse, slightly concave at the bottom, and four to six centimetres long; its mid-point lies on the ascending path of the previously identified trunk of the VSE. The subcutaneous cellular tissue, which is often extensive in women, is cut transversely down to the aponeurosis over a radius of three to five centimetres (). A five-centimetre longitudinal aponevrotomy is performed over the cellulo-adiputic tissue of the popliteal fossa. The ESV must be identified, bearing in mind that it is the most superficial vascular and neural element in the popliteal fossa, usually in contact with the deep surface of the lateral edge of the aponeurosis incised beforehand. Giacomini's vein can be a valuable Ariadne's thread. Proximal dissection of the VSE is then undertaken with scissors and a raised pad (); all the collaterals can be successively tied before sectioning. A common trunk may be found between the ESV and the gastrocnemius vein, which must then be freed until it ends in the popliteal vein. The wall of the VSE at its termination is generally quite thin and fragile and must be dissected with care. The end of the ESV is not necessarily located on the posterior surface of the popliteal vein. It may be posterolateral or anterolateral, or more exceptionally anterior. The VSE is approached at its origin by a short, one-centimetre transverse cutaneous incision at the level of the fossa defined by the posterior edge of the external malleolus and the calcaneal tendon. The vein is in the subcutaneous cellular tissue. It is depressible, of supple consistence and should not be confused with the external saphdna nerve fascicle, pearly ivory, of firmer consistence, which is 6troitely accolë. The approach to the VSE in its leg course is facilitated by the prëopëratory ëchographic repërage. The lower two-thirds of the incision is subcuticular and can therefore be easily approached via a posterior median incision of two to three centimetres. In its proximal third, the RipoiK'vrose must be incised; the VSE is easily found in contact with the deep surface of the latter.

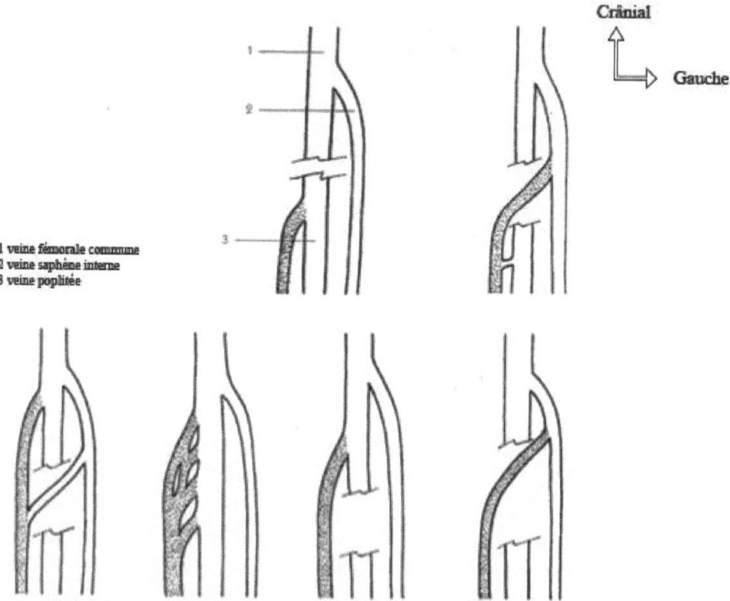

Figure 19: termination modes of the VSE, shown in grey on the drawings.

5.2.2.1.3- Indications:

5.2.2.1.3.1- Thoracic pathologies :

Pleural effusion :

- Treatment of the condition causing pleural effusion
- Drainage of large pleural ëpanches.

The drainage technique [35] :

a) Installation of the patient In all cases, the patient is installed in dorsal dëcubitus, with the arm homolatëral to the lesion abducted or even behind the head to expose the axillary fossa. The necessary equipment must be placed on a sterile tray and in particular the trocars, drains, connectors and tubes must be checked before starting the anaesthetic.

b) Asepsis Pleural drainage is an invasive procëdure involving insertion of a drain for several days. Aseptic insertion is essential to limit the risk of infection of the operative site and pleural empyëme.

c) L Eiuilgesia Thoracic drainage is a painful procedure. In the conscious patient on spontaneous ventilation, local anaesthetic is rëalisëe a few minutes before drain insertion combined with parenteral analgesia (paracetamol, nefopam, morphine). The eventuality of a vagal malaise when the drain is inserted or during re-expansion of the lung must be anticipated.

d) Drainage approaches The axillary route: The puncture zone is delimited by the safety triangle. This triangle is defined at the back by the posterior axillary line, at the bottom by the level of the nipple (5th intercostal space) and at the front by the posterior edge of the pectoralis major. The point of insertion corresponds to the 4th intercostal space on the anterior or middle axillary line. The main risk is of draining too far down, which could damage the diaphragmatic dome and the underlying intra-abdominal organs. Theoretically, this is the best way to drain a pleural fluid effusion.

The anterior route: This is located on the mid-clavicular line at the level of the 2nd intercostal space. If the drainage is too internal, there is a risk of blocking the internal mammary artery. The disadvantage is that the pectoralis major muscle is damaged and the scars are very unaesthetic. It is шШзёе in the drainage of a hëmothorax in the polytraumatisë and ventilated patient.

e) Insertion of the drain A 2 cm incision of the intercostal space is rëalisëe at the level of the superior border of the infëternal side. The wall is dissected plane by plane using Kelly's forceps. The opening of the parietal lip is rëalisëe with forceps. The pleura may be explored using a finger to feel the lung and check for adhesions. The drain is introduced into the pleural space apically to drain a pneumothorax and posterobasally to drain a hemothorax. Progression of the drain into the pleural space is stopped when Ыдёге resistance is perceived. Once in place, the drain is connected to a drainage system. The position of the drain must always be checked by a control X-ray.

Respiratory kinesitherapy [35]: This is the other essential aspect of the management of thoracic trauma. The aim is to improve drainage of tracheobronchial secretions and inspiratory function, thereby optimising hematosis and reducing the incidence of atelectasis. Positive pressure ventilation is used for alveolar recruitment. The discovery of atelectasis or the occurrence of significant bronchial congestion should prompt consideration of either postural drainage (delicate in the case of rib fractures) or bronchoaspiration under fibroscopy.

Pericarditis [21] :

Medical treatment :

Painkillers and anti-inflammatories are enough to reduce the inflammation in most cases. If, however, there is a large accumulation of fluid, the situation may be critical for the patient. The cardiologist then urgently ëvacuates the fluid by inserting a small catheter into the pericardial cavity. The small device is placed for a period varying from a few hours to a few days, until the excessive production of the fluid stops. **Surgical treatment :**

Surgical treatment is the last resort if the indication is posëe.

Firm chest trauma [22] :

Medical treatment :

The main aims of medical treatment are to re-establish correct oxygenation and good blood flow, relieve pain and prevent superinfection.

Resuscitation:

In the majority of cases, the usual means of resuscitation are l'охудёпайоп, vascular filling and blood transfusion. These measures are generally sufficient.

Anaesthesia Treatment of the pain associated with thoracic trauma is the mainstay of medical treatment. Minor analgesics (paracetamol) are used routinely. Morphine can be used in boluses.

Antibiotic prophylaxis aims to prevent infection of skin wounds and drainage sites.

Instrumental means Essentially evacuating pleural puncture allowing decompression before drainage in very large effusions.

Surgical treatment :

Surgical treatment Patient consent and information It is desirable to explain the procedure and its risks to the patient. In the event of an emergency, this information is différëe.

Pleural drainage [11, 26] Thoracic drainage or pleural drainage is performed by introducing a drain into the pleural space to ëvacuate any ëhemorrhagic or gaseous effusion. This re-establishes a negative pressure in the pleural cavity to bring the surface of the lung back to the chest wall.

Pleural drainage is aimed at emptying effusions and holding the lung to the wall; monitoring bleeding by measuring the hourly flow rate; evacuating blood and clots to reduce the risk of secondary infection.

Endothoracic goitres [22] :

Medical treatment :

Treatment varies according to the cause and severity of the goitre. The goitre may remain small, without influencing hormone secretion or creating compression. In this case, regular endocrinological monitoring is suggested, including palpation, ultrasound and blood tests.

Surgical treatment :

Surgical treatment is indicated for very unpleasant or annoying goitres in the neck area, leading to hyperthyroidism. The operation involves complete or partial removal of the gland (thyroidectomy).

When the goitre extends down the trachea and invades the chest, it is known as an endothoracic (or plunging) goitre. Surgical treatment is then proposed, usually involving an incision in the neck (cervicotomy) or, if necessary, an opening in the sternum (sternotomy).

Diaphragmatic hernias [22] :

The treatment is surgical repair.

5.2.2.1.3.2-   Vascular pathologies :

Arteriopathies :

Medical Treatment

Atheromatous arteriopathy of the lower limbs:

If left untreated, this disease, which is considered serious, can lead to **disabling conditions, including amputation [23]**. It also **considerably reduces life expectancy**. It is also **a warning sign** that may conceal a cardiovascular ëкyë risk.

The treatment is based on **lifestyle measures** such as quitting smoking, losing weight if necessary, daily exercise and a balanced diet.

Medication is administered. It includes :

*   **An antiplatelet agent** to thin the blood so that it does not form clots in the artery;
*   **An ACE inhibitor** which protects the arteries from the effects of atheroma;
*   **A statin** to control cholestërol;

Arteriopathy of the upper limbs [14] :

Treatment is based on **corticotherapy.**

Surgical treatment

Surgery should **only be performed in emergency situations.** If it fails, or if the situation is serious, **revascularisation** (dilatation and/or stenting, bypass surgery) or amputation should be performed.

Arteriovenous fistulas [25] :
AVF is performed during a surgical procedure that involves connecting an artery and a vein in the forearm or upper arm. This makes it possible to significantly increase the blood flow in a superficial vein, a prerequisite for easy puncture and obtaining a sufficient quantity of blood for the **dialysis machine.**
The major advantage of the **arteriovenous fistula** is that it can be used for several years, and has a low infection rate.
Where is the arteriovenous fistula performed? [25] :
In a дёпёгаlе manner, the **AVF** will be placëe to the forearm or arm. The vascular surgeon will favour **the non-dominant arm** so as not to disrupt the patient's daily routine. It is proximal or distal
- The left arm for right-handed people
- The right arm for left-handed people

Deep vein thrombosis [27] :
Treatments for phlebitis are aimed at relieving symptoms and preventing further clots from forming. It may be necessary to remove the clot or inject drugs to dissolve it. The doctor may also prescribe anticoagulant injections or oral medication, as well as compression stockings. Sometimes, in the event of a recurrence in a superficial vein, the doctor may have the affected vein removed. Immobilisation should be for as short a time as possible, and activities should be resumed gradually.
Compression stockings must be worn for at least two years for proximal deep vein thrombosis and 6 months for distal DVT.
It is important to adhere to the medicinal and non-medicinal treatments prescribed by your doctor for the full recommended duration.
Elastic support is an essential element in the prevention and treatment of venous thrombosis. It consists of wearing socks, knee-highs, stockings and tights that exert pressure on the leg, which, with movement, encourages blood to circulate in the veins and rise towards the heart.
Compression stockings (sometimes called **varicose stockings**) are divided into three classes according to the pressure they exert on the leg, expressed in millimetres of mercury (mmHg):
- **Class I stockings** exert a pressure of 10 to 15 mm Hg. They are best suited to people who stand for long periods, pregnant women, long-distance travellers and those suffering from venous insufficiency;
- **Class II" stockings** exert a pressure of 15 to 20 mm Hg. They are prescribed for people who have just undergone vein surgery, pregnant women and travellers at particular risk of venous thrombosis, as well as for people with varicose veins or swelling (redemas) of the legs;
- **Class III" stockings** exert a pressure of 20 to 36 mm Hg. They are intended for people with a history of venous thrombosis and those suffering from severe varicose veins, severe leg swelling or post-thrombotic syndrome.
There are stronger compression stockings (30 to 40 mm Hg) which seem particularly useful for preventing post-thrombotic syndrome.
Compression stockings **are contraindicated** for diabetics suffering from severe disorders of the small blood vessels (microangiopathy), for people with arterial disease of the legs (arteritis), and for those with loss of feeling in the feet and legs (neuropathy) or untreated heart failure.
There are different **sizes of** compression stockings. The pharmacist should measure the ankle

in the morning to determine the correct stocking size. The choice between socks, stockings or tights depends on the location of the thrombosis.

Venous insufficiency :

Treatment [28] :

• Venous support, in the form of stockings or elastic bands wrapped around the limb, promotes venous return, relieves leg heaviness and reduces redemes. It is contraindicated in cases of severe arteriopathy of the limbs.

• Pharmacological treatment: of modest effectiveness, "venotonics" can be used occasionally, in addition to compression therapy, particularly in the warmer months when clinical signs are more severe (and compression therapy more painful).

• Sclerotherapy: may be indicated for superficial venous insufficiency when the largest trunks (saphenous veins) are not severely affected. It is most often proposed for aesthetic purposes.

Surgical treatment :

Interventional treatment: using conventional surgery (or cryotherapy) or the endo-laser method, the aim is to remove diseased segments of superficial veins. In this case, venous return is exclusively via the deep veins. It is therefore essential to ensure that these veins are patent.

compartment syndromes [29] :

Medical treatment :

Medical treatment is based on probabilistic antibiotic therapy before and after surgery, before obtaining an antibiogram and introducing the appropriate antibiotic. Painkillers and low molecular weight anticoagulants are also required, as well as elevation of the limb to promote venous return.

Surgical treatment :

The treatment is aponevrotomy.

IV- Patients and method

IV.1- Setting and place of study :

This work was carried out in the thoracic and cardiovascular surgery department "Andre FESTOC centre" at the Mëre- Enfant le "Luxembourg" hospital centre in Bamako.

The Mère - Enfant "Luxembourg" hospital centre in Bamako is a second-tier private healthcare establishment in Mali's health pyramid.

It is home to a diverse population from all over the country and the West African sub-region.

The Andre FESTOC centre is one of the leading centres for thoracic and cardiovascular surgery in Mali.

The introduction of a new medical speciality always creates the risk of delimiting its field of activity, as it is always done by dismembering a pre-existing speciality. The thoracic and vascular surgery unit has taken on patients from these specialities over a long and gradual period. It has taken over activities previously carried out in ENT, general surgery, orthopaedic traumatology, cancerology, pneumology and cardiology.

With the gradual increase in the number of patients treated over the years, there has been a clear improvement. At present, the field of thoracic surgery encompasses mainly pleuropulmonary, parietal and mediastinal surgery. The frontier areas are still disputed between it and ENT on the one hand and visceral surgery on the other. There are fewer conflicts in vascular surgery, but the management of diabetic feet is still shared between vascular surgery and orthopaedics, which makes it difficult to adopt a unified approach to patients. The same applies to vascular trauma. The Cardiovascular Thoracic Surgery Department did not exist at the ME University Hospital until August 2018, so activity was erratic and patients were operated on in different, distant departments where the necessary infrastructure and staff were not always optimised.

Nursing staff had to be trained several times to get them used to this type of patient. They had to be taught how to monitor thoracic drainage, how to use anticoagulants sensibly, and the indications for thoracic and vascular pathologies. There is an urgent need for investment to ensure that the minimum conditions are in place for this type of surgery to continue to develop.

Thoracic and vascular surgery requires specialised medical and paramedical staff, as well as consultation, surgical and hospital facilities adapted to these specialities.

The Andre FESTOC centre includes :

- Two operating theatres, one dedicated to cardiac surgery and the other to thoracic and vascular surgery;
- A 6-bed intensive care unit, including an isolation room;
- A decontamination and sterilisation room;
- A pharmacy room ;
- A staff duty room and a refectory;
- Two changing rooms for men and women;
- Two surgery consultation offices;
- An anaesthesia and intensive care unit;
- An adult and paediatric inpatient unit;
- A biomedical workshop;

- A consumable storage room;
- A dressing room (outpatients) ;
- An archive room ;
- A staff room.

4.1.1- The staff includes :
- Two thoracic and cardiovascular surgeons, all masters of research;
- Four anaesthetists, including 2 senior lecturers;
- Four cardiologists, including one of magisterial rank, one lecturer and one research fellow;
- Three perfusionists, including 2 autonomous perfusionists;
- Five doctoral students working as interns and students specialising in cardiology, thoracic and cardiovascular surgery, anaesthesia and intensive care are on rotation;
- Paramedical staff (operating theatre, intensive care, hospitalisation, consultation, treatment room) and support staff;
- Six service maintenance staff ;

4.1.2- How the service works :

Hospital activities take up a large part of the time of these medical and paramedical staff. This does not mean that the academic function suffers too much, as the department's workload is clearly defined.
- Hospital admissions ;
- Outpatient consultations (new and old patients)
- Medical and surgical treatment ;
- Training for medical and paramedical students

4.1.3- Hospital admissions :

Types of patients to be hospitalised :
- Emergencies: these are patients from other departments (cardiology, orthopaedics, traumatology, medicine, paediatrics, pneumology, oncology, nephrology, etc.) who come under our speciality, patients seen on an outpatient basis and whose case requires hospitalisation.
- Non-emergency cases: these are cases hospitalised by appointment.

Hospitalisation is therefore carried out at any time for the first group and only the day before the operation for the second group.

4.1.4- Consultations :

They are available Monday to Friday from 08:00 to 16:00 for seniors and emergencies 7 days a week.

4.1.5- Medical and surgical treatment :

4.1.5.1-   Medical treatment :

It is used in association with surgical treatment or, better still, as a framework for the treatment of clinical manifestations that require surgical intervention.

As we can see, the service is part of a complex. Its operation is coordinated, but above all it is subordinate to the complex in both qualitative and quantitative terms.

However, it should be noted that in some cases the diagnostic and therapeutic procedures are complementary with those of other departments at the **CHU-ME.**

Close collaboration between these groups is essential if these complementary disciplines are to be more efficient and effective.

4.1.5.2- Surgical treatment :

These are conditions relating to surgery for thoracic and vascular pathologies.

IV.2- Type of study :

This was a retrospective and descriptive study carried out at the Andre FESTOC Centre of the "Luxembourg" University Hospital in Bamako (CHUME-B). It focused on the records of patients who had been treated for thoracic and/or vascular pathology in the department during the study period.

IV.3- Period of study :

The study was dëroulëe over a përiode of five (5) years from 1er January 2018 to 31 dëcembre 2022.

IV.4- Study population :

This study concerned all patients managed for thoracic or vascular pathology operated on or not at the Andre FESTOC centre of the university hospital centre Mëre- enfant le "Luxembourg" in Bamako (CHUME-B).

IV.5- Inclusion criteria :

The study included :

- All patients referred or having consulted for thoracic and vascular pathology;
- Operated and non-operated patients;
- Any patient whose file was complete;

IV.6- Non-inclusion criteria :

Not included in this study:

- Patients treated for pure cardiac pathology ;
- Patients whose files were incomplete;
- Patients treated elsewhere outside the Andre Festoc centre

IV.7- Data support :

Data were collected from patients' consultation records, hospital admissions and operative reports. These data were compiled on a questionnaire drawn up by ourselves, corrected by the co-director and validated by the thesis director. It included data relating to sociodëmographic parameters, the clinic, therapeutic management, etc.

IV.8- Data capture and analysis :

Data were collected and entered using Microsoft World and Excel 2016. Data processing and analysis were performed using SPSS version 25 statistical software, $P < 0.05$ is significant.

IV.9- Ethical considerations :

We obtained the patients' consent, and confidentiality was respected.

IV.10- Gantt chart

Digram of Garret					
Periods	**University Years 2022- 2023**				
Activities	**June2022- July 2022**	**July 2022 - august2022**	**August2022- sept2022**	**October 2022 -March 20223**	**April 2023 -May2023**	**May2023 June 2023**
Review of literature	X					
Drawing up the questionnaire		X				
Mask for data entry			X			
Investigation of				XXXXXX		

files						
Data capture, processing and analysis					X	
Writing the thesis						X

V- Results

V.1- Overall frequency :

Over 5 years, the thoracic and vascular surgery department recorded 1,720 consultations, including 581 patients suffering from thoracic pathology and 1,139 patients for vascular pathology. A total of 792 surgical procedures were performed, including 402 thoracic procedures and 390 vascular procedures.

Thoracic pathologies accounted for 33.78% of consultations and 66.22% for vascular pathologies. The department's surgical activity rose by 46.04%. Thoracic pathologies accounted for 50.75% of surgical procedures and 49.25% for vascular surgery.

V.2- Epidemiological aspects :

V.2.1- Breakdown by revolution of the overall number of patients per year

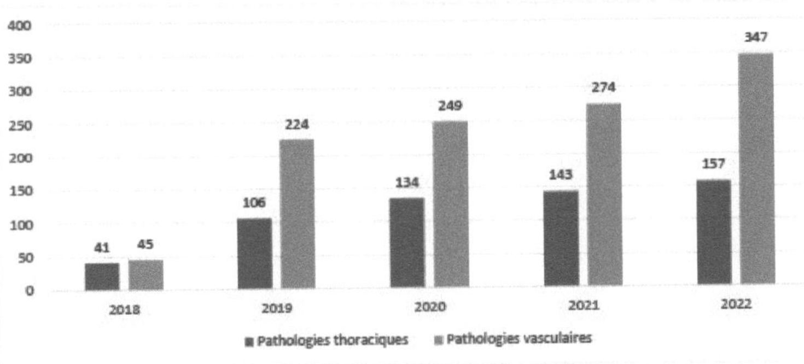

Figure 20: Overall distribution of patients according to Involution of care per year.

The number of patients cared for has gradually increasedë over the years to reach 157 thoracic pathology patients and 347 vascular pathology patients in 2022.

V.2.2- Distribution according to overall patient age :

Table I: Age distribution of patients.

Age (years)	Workforce	Percentages (%)
0-15	75	4,40
16 - 30	194	11,30
31 - 45	334	19,4
46 - 60	496	28,90
61 - 75	448	26
>76	173	10
Total	**1720**	**100,00**

The overall mean age of the patients was 51.34 years, with a standard deviation of 19.51 and [2 months and 123 years].

V.2.3- **Gender distribution of patients :**

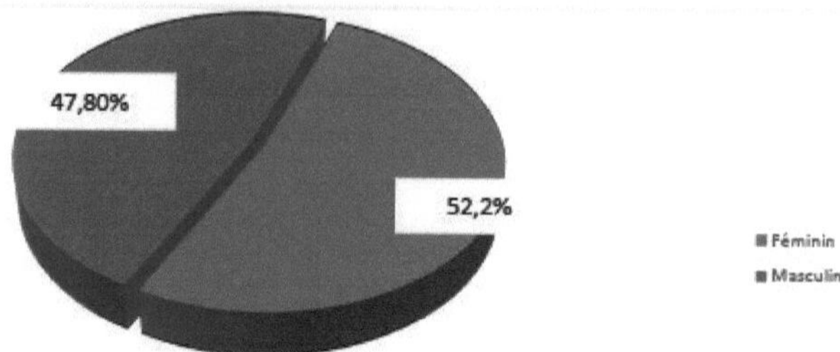

Figure 21: Overall distribution of patients by gender.

The overall sex ratio was 0.91.

5.2.3 **Breakdown by overall patient origin :**

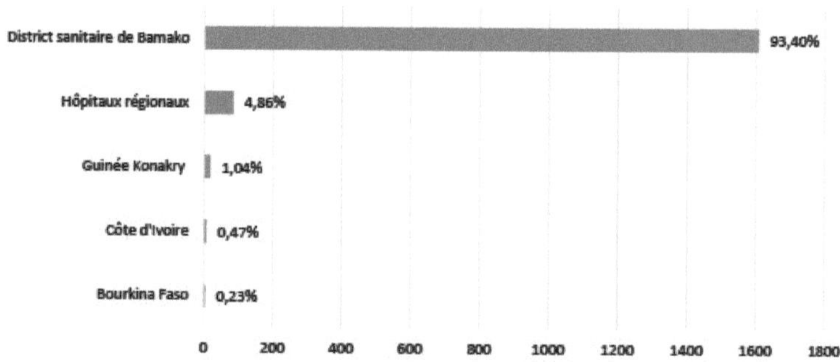

Figure 22: Overall distribution of patients according to origin.

The overall majority of patients (93.40%) came from the Bamako district.

5.2.4 **Breakdown of patients by main occupation :**

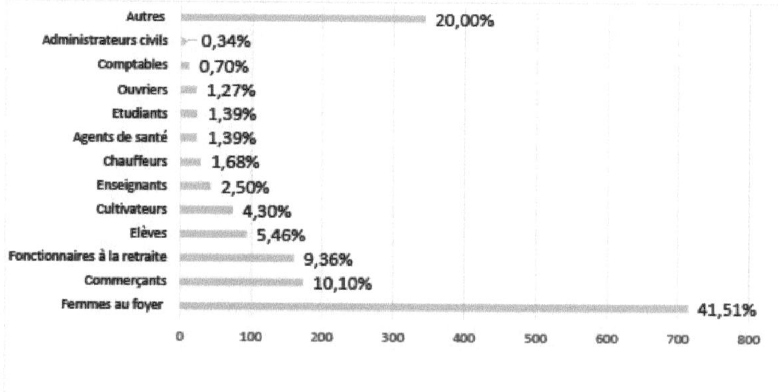

Figure 23: Overall distribution of patients according to their main occupations.

Housewives were the most represented with 41.51%.

5.3 **Breakdown by nosological group :**

The affectons taken care of were ële divided into 2 groups:

40

Thoracic and vascular pathologies.

5.3.1- Thoracic pathologies :

A total of 581 patients, or 33.78% of consultations, were analysed according to age, sex, diagnosis, treatment and immëdiate results.

5.3.1.1- Age distribution of thoracic surgery patients :

Table II: Rëpartition of patients by age in thoracic surgery.

Age (years)	Workforce	Percentages (%)
0 - 15	52	9
16 - 30	94	16,17
31-45	123	21,03
46- 60	167	29
61-75	118	20,30
>76	27	4,50
Total	**581**	**100,00**

The mean age of thoracic surgery patients ëwas 44.65 years with a ëstandard deviation of 20.26 and [from 2 months to 94 years].

5.3.1.2- Gender distribution of thoracic surgery patients :

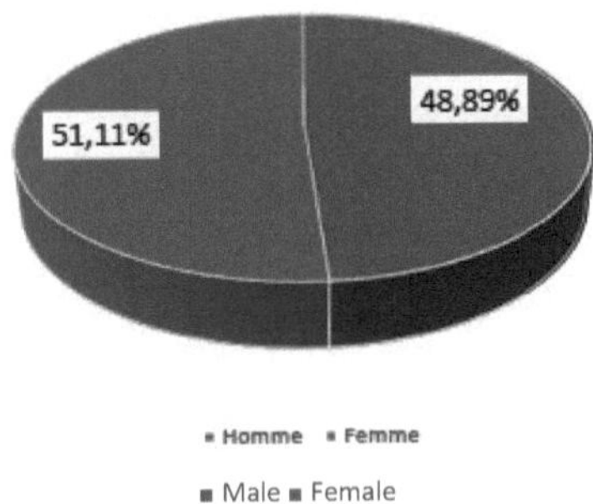

Figure 24: Rëpartition of thoracic pathology patients by gender.

The sex ratio ël ɯ1: of 0.95 in thoracic pathology.

5.3.1.3- Breakdown by main occupation in thoracic surgery :

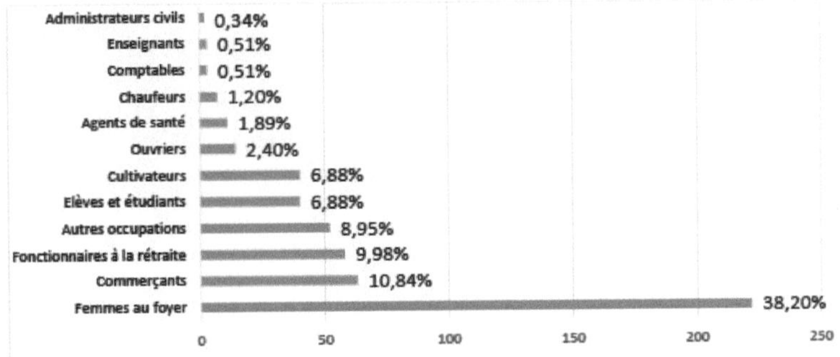

Figure 25: Rëpartition of patients according to main occupation in thoracic surgery. Housewives accounted for the majority of patients, with 38.20% in thoracic pathology.

5.3.1.4- Breakdown by origin of thoracic pathology patients:

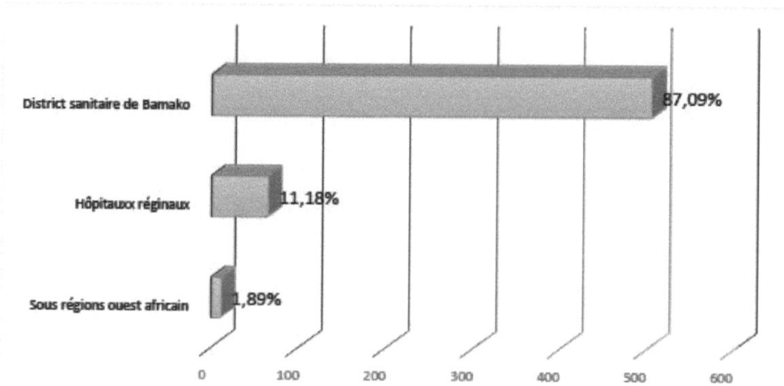

Figure 26: Breakdown of patients by thoracic pathology origin.

87.09% of thoracic pathology patients were from the Bamako district.

5.3.1.5- Breakdown by type of thoracic pathology :

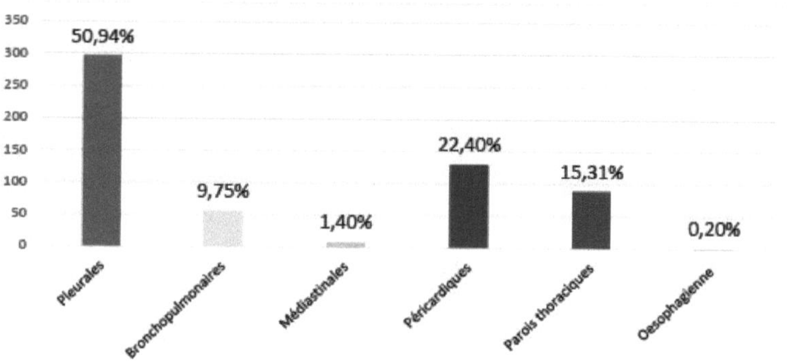

Figure 27: Distribution of patients according to type of thoracic pathology.

5.3.1.6-

Pleural, përicardial and chest wall pathologies were the main pathologies observed, with 50.94%, 22.40%, and 15.31% in thoracic pathology respectively.

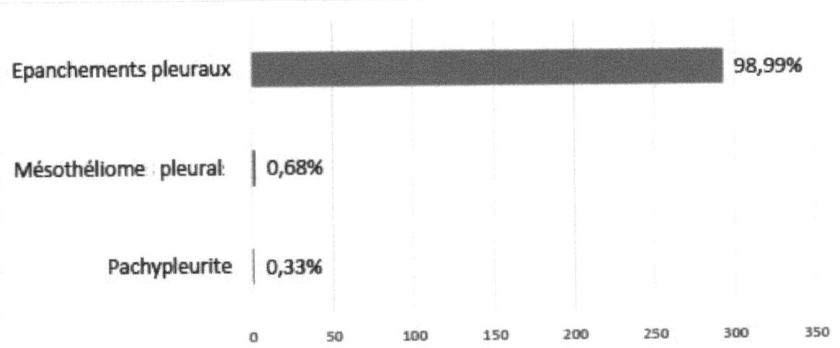

5.3.1.7- Breakdown by type of pleural pathology :

Figure 28: Distribution of patients by type of pleural pathology.

Pleural effusions accounted for 98.99% of pleural pathologies.

5.3.1.8- Breakdown by type of pleural effusion :

Table III: Rëpartition of patients according to type of pleural effusion.

Type	Workforce	Percentage (%)
Pleuresie	160	81,63
Pneumothorax	28	14,28
Mixed effusion	8	4,09
Total	**196**	**100,00**

Pleural effusions accounted for 81.63% of all pleural effusions.

5.3.1.9- Breakdown by type of bronchopulmonary pathology :

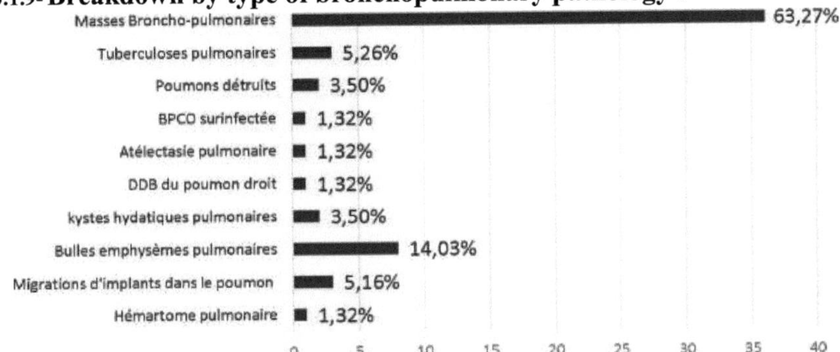

Figure 29: Breakdown of patients by type of bronchopulmonary disease.

Malignant bronchopulmonary masses accounted for 63.27%.

5.3.1.10- Depending on the location of the bronchopulmonary mass in the thorax:

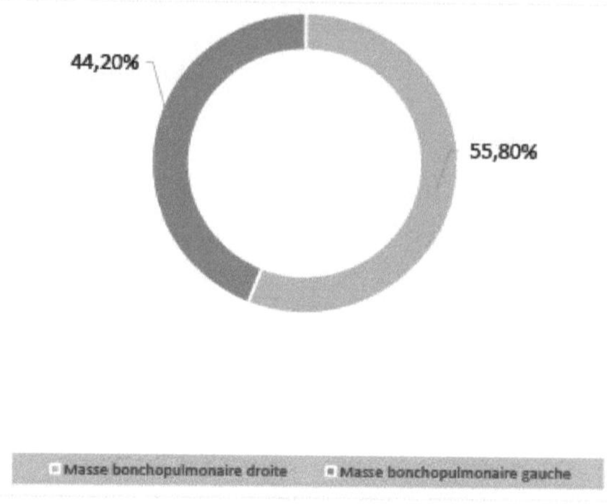

[Right bonchopulmonary mass "Left bonchopulmonary mass

Figure 30: Distribution of patients according to the location of the bronchopleural mass.

In more than half the patients (55.80%), the bronchopulmonary mass was located on the right.

5.3.1.11- Distribution according to mediastinal pathologies :

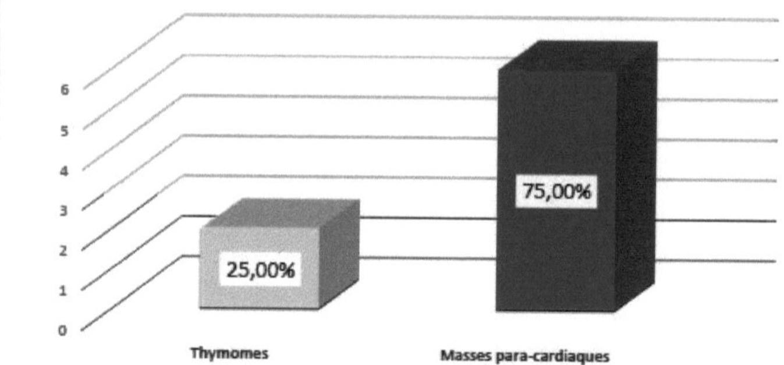

Figure 31: Distribution of patients according to mediastinal pathology.

In most cases, it was a paracardiac mass (75.00% of cases).

5.3.1.12- Distribution according to the type of pericardial effusion :

Table IV: Rëpartition of patients according to the type of përicardial embolism.

Type of effusion	Workforce	Percentage (%)
Acute përicardial effusion	97	74,61
Pleuropëricardial effusion	23	17,69
Chronic constructive përicardial effusion	10	7,70
Total	**130**	**100,00**

Acute heart attacks accounted for 74.61%.

5.3.1.13-   **Distribution according to chest wall pathologies :**

Table *V*: Rëpartition of patients according to chest wall pathologies.

Chest wall disorders	Workforce	Percentage (%)
Abcës pariëtal	1	1,75
Adënite thoracic reaction	1	1,75
Supernumerary breast	1	1,75
Post-fracture callus of the right clavicle	1	1,75
Parietal pain	1	1,75
Thoracic paravertebral neuroma	1	1,75
Breast cancer	4	7,01
Pariëtal weights	12	21,05
Trauma to the chest	35	61,44
Total	**57**	**100,00**

Thoracic fermës trauma accounted for 61.44% followed by pariëtal mass in 21.05% of cases.

5.3.1.14-   **Breakdown by mechanism of thoracic trauma :**

Table VI: Rëpartition of patients by type of thoracic trauma.

Type of trauma	Workforce	Percentage (%)
Traumatic stroke	32	91,42
Ballistic trauma	2	5,71
Blunt force trauma	1	2,85
Total	**35**	**100,00**

91.42% of closed chest injuries were secondary to an MVA.

5.3.1.15-   **Distribution according to esophageal pathology :**

- Only one patient was treated for cancer of the 1'resophagus.

5.3.1.16-   **Distribution according to other thoracic pathologies treated :**

Table VII: Rëpartition of patients according to other pathologies.

Other pathologies	Workforce	Percentage (%)
Dëformations of the thorax	4	12,12
Hëpatic abcës	3	9,10
Endothoracic goitres	14	42,42
Chest pain	1	3,03
Diaphragmatic hernias	11	33,33
Total	**33**	**100,00**

The most frequent pathologies at the thoracic frontiëres ëtaient endothoracic goitres (42.42%) followed by diaphragmatic hernias (33.33%).

5.3.2- Vascular pathologies :

With 1139 patients consulted, vascular pathologies represented a significant proportion of the department's activities. Patient numbers have risen sharply over the last three years.

5.3.2.1- Age distribution of vascular surgery patients :

Table *VIII*: Age distribution of vascular surgery patients.

Age (years)	Workforce	Percentages (%)
0 - 15	23	2,01
16 - 30	100	8,77
31 - 45	211	18,30
46 - 60	329	29,14
61 - 75	330	28,97
>76	146	12,81
Total	**1139**	100,00

The mean age of vascular pathology patients was 54.60 years, with a standard deviation of 18.24 and extremes of 3 and 123 years.

5.3.2.2- Gender distribution of vascular surgery patients :

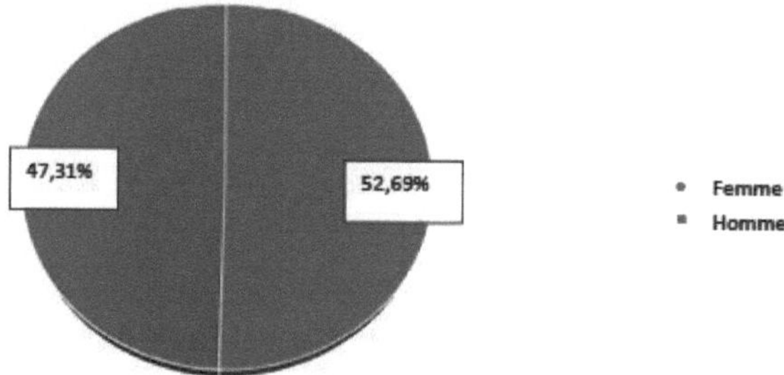

Figure 32: Gender distribution of vascular surgery patients.

The sex ratio of vascular surgery patients was 0.89.

5.3.2.3- Breakdown by main occupation of vascular surgery patients :

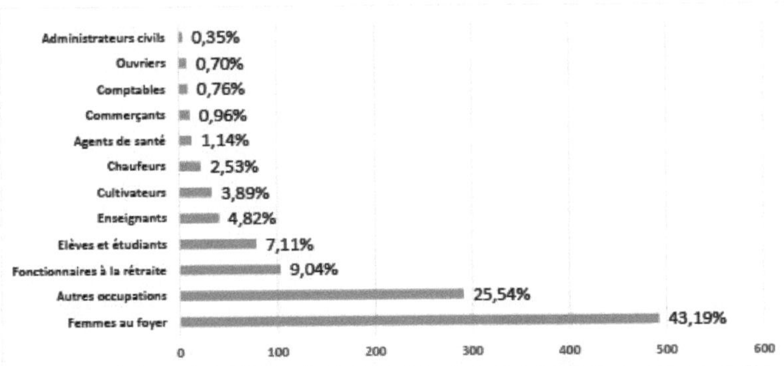

Figure 33: Rëpartition of patients by main occupation in vascular surgery. Housewives dominated the vascular surgery sample with 43.19% of cases.

5.3.2.4- Breakdown by origin of vascular pathology patients.

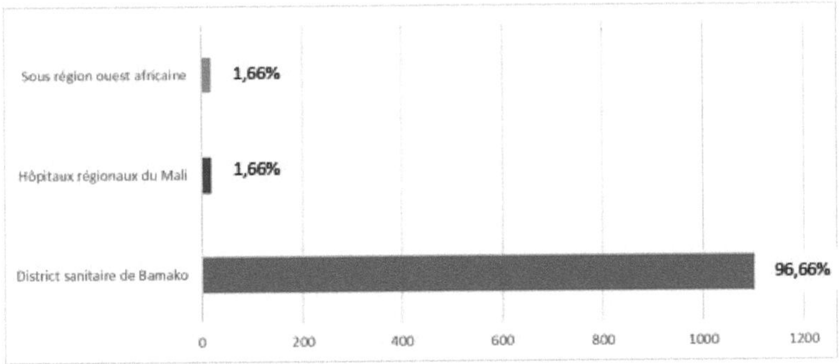

Figure 34: Rëpartition of patients by vascular surgery origin.

The majority of patients came from the Bamako district, accounting for 96.66% of cases.

5.3.2.5- Breakdown by type of vascular pathology :

Pathologies associated with vascular pathologies

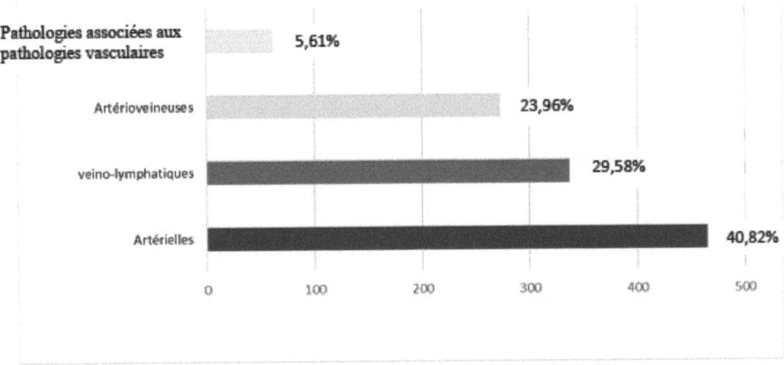

Figure 35: Distribution of patients by type of vascular pathology.

Arterial pathologies accounted for 40.82% of cases.

5.3.2.6- Distribution according to location of arterial disease :

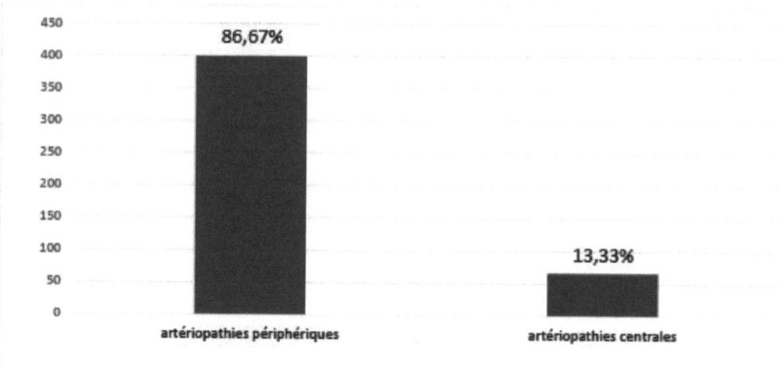

Figure 36 : Distribution of patients by location of arterial disease

86.67% of arteriopathies had a peripheral location in vascular pathology.

Table IX: Distribution of patients according to the type of përiphëric arteriopathy.

Type of arteriopathyStrength	Percentage (%)
Arteriopathy of the limbs366	90,81
Stenosis of the carotid artery26	6,46
Arterial thrombosis11	2,73
Total403	**100,00**

Limb aiteriopathy was present in 90.81% of cases.

5.3.2.6- Distribution according to location of aneurysmal pathology :

Table X: Rëpartition of patients according to the location of the aortic aneurysm.

LocationStaff	Percentage (%)
Abdominal aorta16	38,10
Thoracoabdominal aorta15	35,71
Thoracic aorta8	19,04
Aortic arch3	7,15
Total42	**100,00**

The aneurysm was located in the abdominal aorta in 38.10% of cases, followed by a thoraco-abdominal location in 35.71% of cases.

Table XI: Distribution of patients according to the peripheral arterial location of the aneurysm.

Peripheral locationStaff	Percentage (%)
Right subclavian artery2	33,32
Left vertebral artery1	16,67
Left superficial femoral artery1	16,67
Deep femoral artery1	16,67

| Mega TABC1 | 16,67 |
| **Total6** | **100,00** |

Aneurysm of the right subclavian artery was the most frequent peripheral location with 33.32%.

5.3.2.7- Distribution according to the type of arterial dissection :

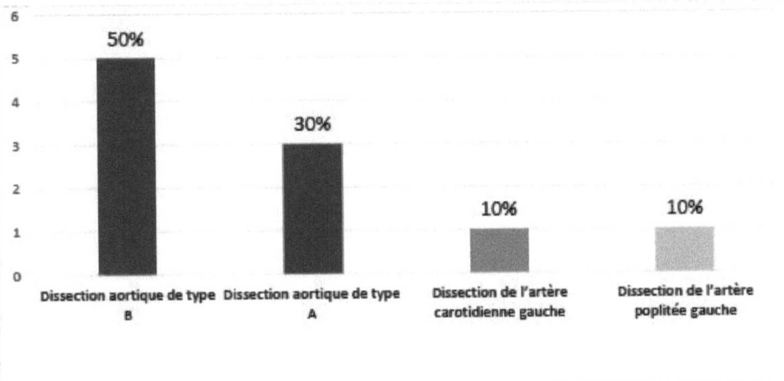

Figure 37: Rëpartition of patients according to the type of arterial dissection.

Type B aortic dissection was common, accounting for 50% of all dissections.

5.3.2.8- Other arterial pathologies

> **Horton's disease :**

Two patients had Ьёпёйаё temporal artery biopsy for histologically confirmedë Horton's disease.

> **Arterial malformations**

1 patient had an unoperated Arteria Lusoria

5.3.2.9- Breakdown by type of veno-lymphatic pathology :

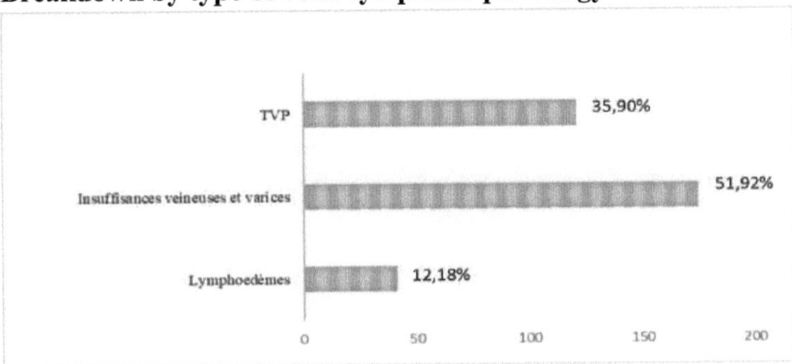

Figure 38: Rëpartition of patients by type of veno-lymphatic pathology.

Venous insufficiency and DVT dominated veno-lymphatic pathology with 51.92% and 35.95% respectively.

5.3.2.10- **Depending on the location of the deep vein thrombosis :**

Table XII: Breakdown of patients by DVT location

Location	Workforce	Percentage (%)
Pelvic limbs	111	91,73
Thoracic limbs	7	5,79
Internal jugular veins	3	2,48
Total	121	100,00

DVT was localised to the pelvic limbs in 91.73 of patients.

5.3.2.11- **Distribution according to topography of deep vein thrombosis in the pelvic limbs :**

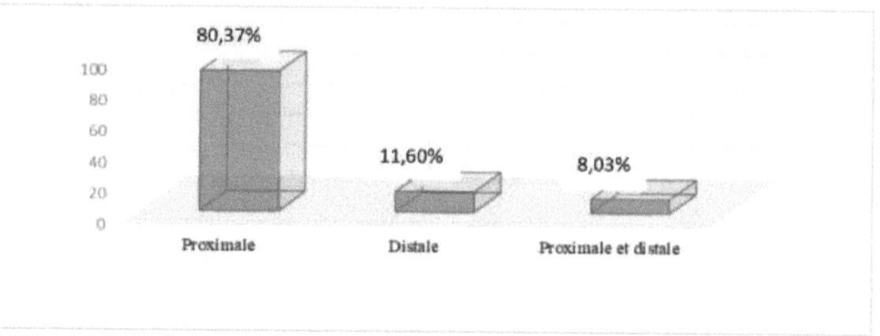

Figure 39: Rëpartition of patients by topography of DVT to pelvic limbs.

80.37% of pelvic limb DVTs ëtended to be proximal.

5.3.2.12- **Breakdown by type of venous insufficiency :**

Table XIII: Rëpartition according to the type of venous insufficiency.

Venous insufficiency type	Workforce	Percentage (%)
Bilateral DVI	73	41,71
Unilateral CVI	48	27,43
Varicose veins	54	30,86
Total	175	100,00

Varicose veins were diagnosed in 30.86% of patients as a complication of chronic venous insufficiency.

5.3.2.13- **Breakdown by type of varicose vein :**

Table XIV: Breakdown of patients by type of varicose vein.

Type	Workforce	Percentage (%)
Varicose veins GVS	15	27,78
Varicose vein PVS	5	9,25
Bilateral varicose vein GVS	25	46,30
икёге varicose veins	8	14,81
Varicose vein rupture during pregnancy	1	1,86
Total	54	100,00

The varicose vein was complicated by varicose ulcëre in 14.81% of patients.

 Distribution according to lymphaden location:

Table XV: Distribution of patients according to the type of lymphaemia.

Type	Workforce	Percentage (%)
Primary	36	87,80
Secondary	5	12,20
Total	41	100,00

In 87.80% of patients it was a primary lymphaemia.

Table XVI: Distribution of patients according to the location of the primary lymphaemia.

Location	Workforce	Percentage (%)
Biateraie MI	14	38,89
Uniiateraie MI	22	61,11
Total	**36**	**100,00**

Primary lymphredemas ëtaient unilateraux dans 61,11% des cas. Secondary lymphadenemas ëtaient iocaiisës aux membres thoraciques et consëcutifs a ia cure chirurgicaie de cancer de sein.

We have recensë 5 cases of patients opërësed for chamber implantation for ia realization of chemiotlierapy.

5.3.2.15- **Arteriovenous pathology :**

> **Arteriovenous fistula for hemodialysis**

Table XVII: Rëpartition of patients according to ia topography of the AVF.

Location of FAV	Workforce	Percentage (%)
Proximaie	140	76,92
Forest	42	23,08
Total	**182**	**100,00**

Proximal AVF was present in 76.92% of renal failure patients.

> **Arteriovenous malformation of the limbs**

- 1 hand AVM
- 3 AVMs in the lower limbs
- 2 Klippei-Trenaunay

5.3.2.17- **Breakdown by type of soft tissue pathology :**

Table XVIII: Rëpartition of patients according to type of soft-tissue pathology.

Type of disease	Workforce	Percentage (%)
Popliteal cyst	4	7,27
Lipoma	4	7,27
Sarcoma	3	5,45
Cheloi'de	1	1,82
Muscle rupture	1	1,82
Nicolau syndrome	1	1,82
Infectious complications	41	74,55
Total	**55**	**100,00**

Soft-tissue infectious complications were the most common in 74.55% of cases.

5.4- Clinical aspects :

5.4.1- Distribution according to risk factors and comorbidities:

Table XIX: Rëpartition of patients according to risk factors and comorbidities in thoracic surgery.

Risk factors	Number (n=581)	Percentage (%)
HTA	164	28,22
Diabetes	99	17,03
Smoking	122	20,99
Asthma	11	1,89
HIV	8	1,37
Hepatitis B	1	0,17
Nephropathy	15	2,58
Heart disease	22	3,78
Tuberculosis	17	2,92
TVP	1	0,17
System disease	5	0,86
Pulmonary embolism	2	0,34
Psychiatric	1	0,17
AVC	4	0,68
Neoplasia	97	16,69

HTA (28.22%), smoking (20.99%), diabëte (17.03%), and nboplasia (16.69% were the main risk factors or comorbidities observed in thoracic surgery.

Table XX: Distribution of patients with risk factors and comorbidities in vascular pathology.

Risk factors in vascular surgery	Number (n=1139)	Percentage (%)
HTA	656	57,59
Diabdte	433	38,01
Smoking	280	24,58
Asthma	4	0,35
HIV	6	0,52
Hepatitis B	2	0,17
Nephropathy	340	29,85
Heart disease	27	2,37
Tuberculosis	1	0,08
TVP	12	1,05
System disease	9	0,79
Pulmonary embolism	7	0,61
Orl sphere infection	14	1,22
Psychiatric	2	0,17
AVC	29	2,54
Neoplasia	18	1,58

Hypertension (57.59%), diabetes (38.01%), kidney disease (29.85%) and smoking (24.58%) were the main risk factors or comorbidities in vascular surgery.

5.4.2- Breakdown by surgical antecedents :

Table XXI: Distribution of patients according to previous thoracic surgery.

Previous thoracic surgery	Number (n=581)	Percentage (%)
Laparotomy	26	4,47
Mastectomy	28	4,81
Limb amputation	5	0,86
Cataract	2	0,34
Thyroi'dectomy	1	0,17
Pericardial drainage	3	0,51
Gynecological	34	5,85
Urological	9	1,54
Thoracotomy	3	0,51
Vascular	6	1,03
Traumatology	23	3,95
Chest drainage	1	0,17
Cardiac	4	0,68
Neurosurgical	9	1,54

Antĕcĕdents from gynaecological surgery (5.85%), mastectomy (4.81%), laparotomy (4 ,47%), and traumatology (3.95%) were most frequently observed in thoracic pathology.

Table XXII: Distribution of patients according to previous vascular surgery.

Previous surgery in vascular surgerySize	(n=1139)	Percentage (%)
Laparotomy	68	5,97
Mastectomy	5	0,43
Limb amputation	32	2,80
Cataract	18	1,58
Thyroi'dectomy	6	0,52
Gynecological	64	5,61
Urological	10	0,87
Vascular	42	3,68
Traumatology	23	2,01
Chest drainage	1	0,80
Cardiac	4	0,35
Neurosurgical	9	0,79

A history of laparotomy surgery (5.97%), gynaecological surgery (5.61%), vascular surgery (3.68%) and limb amputation (2.80%) were most frequently observed in vascular pathology.

5.4.3- Clinical signs of thoracic pathologies :

5.4.3.1- Breakdown by functional signs

Table XXIII: Distribution of patients according to functional signs in thoracic pathologies.

Functional signs	Number (n=581)	Percentage (%)
Chest pain	508	87 ,43
Dyspnea	441	75 ,90
Cough	108	18 ,58
Dysphagia		50,86

Chest pain (87.43%), dyspnoea (75.90%) and cough (18.58%) were the main functional signs observed on admission for thoracic pathology.

5.4.3.1.1- Dyspnea according to the Sadoul scale :

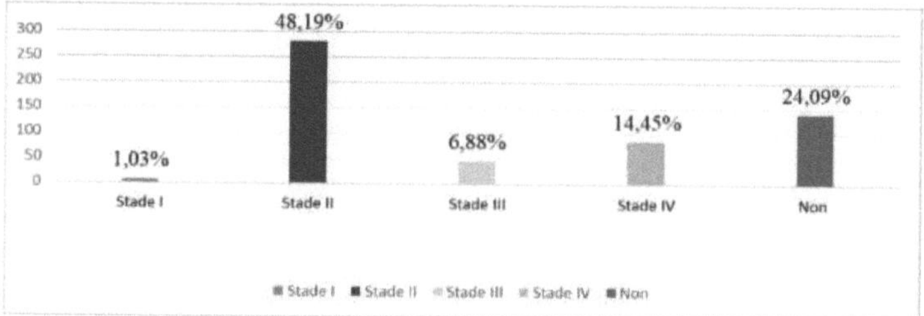

Figure 40: Distribution of patients according to the stage of dyspnea on the Sadoul scale.

Stage II dyspnoea according to the Sadoul scale was frequent on admission in 48.19% of cases, followed by stage IV dyspnoea in 14.45% of cases.

5.4.3.2- Breakdown by physical signs:

Table XXIV: Distribution of patients according to physical signs in thoracic pathology.

Physical signs	Number (n=581)	Percentage (%)
Decreased vesicular murmur	266	45,78
Matite	295	50,77
Reduction in voice vibration	218	37,52
Tympany	77	1,20
Deformation of the thorax	5	0,86

Signs of pleural effusion (50.77%), decreased vesicular murmur (45.78%) and decreased vocal vibration (37.52%) were most frequently observed in thoracic pathology.

5.4.4- Clinical signs of vascular pathologies :

5.4.4.1- Distribution according to functional signs :

Table XXV: Distribution of patients according to functional signs in vascular pathology.

Functional signs	Number (n=1139)	Percentage (%)
Limb pain	1003	88,05
Plantar tingling	269	23,62
Intermittent claudication	272	23,88

Vascular pathologies are most often manifested by pain (88.05%), plantar tingling (23.62%) and intermittent claudication (23.88%) in patients.

Table XXVI: Rëpartition of patients according to përimëtre of walking.

Walking perimeter (m)	Number (n=1139)	Percentage (%)
Normal	669	58,73
<150	470	41,27

The përimëtre de marche was normal in 58.73% of vascular pathology patients.

5.4.4.2- Breakdown by physical signs:

Table XXVII: Rëpartition of patients according to physical signs observed in vascular pathology.

Physical signs	Number (n=1139)	Percentage (%)
Limb swelling	540	47,41
No pulse	465	40,82
Cyanosis	297	26,07
Modification of skin heat	147	12,90
Redness of the limb	54	4,741

Limb tumefaction, absence of pulse and cyanosis were observed with different proportions in vascular pathology: 47.41%, 40.80% and 26.07% respectively.

5.5- Additional tests :

5.5.1- Radiological examinations :

5.5.1.1- Thoracic pathologies :

Table XXVIII: Rëpartition of patients according to complementary examinations rëalisës in thoracic surgery.

Types of examinationStaff (n=581)	Percentage (%)
Chest X-ray498	85,71

Cardiac ultrasound	460	79,17
ECG	413	71,08
Chest scan	163	28,05

Pulmonary X-ray (85.71%), cardiac ultrasound (79.17%), ECG (71.08%) and thoracic CT scan (28.05%) were the most frequently performed complementary examinations in thoracic pathology.

5.5.1.2 Vascular pathologies :

Table XXIX: Rëpartition of patients according to radiological examinations rëalisës in vascular surgery.

Types of examinationStaff (n=1139)	Percentage (%)
Echo-doppler699	61,36
MI, thorax and neck angioscan162	14,22

Doppler and angioscanner were essential examinations in vascular surgery.

5.5.2- Pre-therapeutic biological work-up:

Table XXX: Distribution of patients according to the initial biological work-up carried out in thoracic and vascular surgery.

Biological check-up	Number (N=1720)	Percentage (%)
NFS	839	48,77
CRP	756	43,95
blood lonogram	467	27,15
Transaminases	654	38,02
Creatinine	694	40,34
Uree	512	29,76
TP	609	35,40
TCA	199	11,56
Rhesus grouping	712	41,39

In thoracic and vascular surgery, an initial biological assessment is most often requested.

5.5.3- Other additional biological tests :

Table XXXI: Distribution of patients according to additional biological tests performed.

Supplementary balance sheet	Number (N= 1720)	Percentage (%)
Gen Xpert for biological fluids	195	11,33
Spit BAAR	77	4,53
ECBC	174	10,11
Ag HBS	168	9,76
HCV	165	9,59
HIV	165	9,59
Histology	116	6,74

Depending on the pathology or background, other biological tests may be carried out in addition to the initial biological work-up.

5.6- Therapeutic aspects :

5.6.1 Thoracic diseases :

> **Medical treatment**

Table XXXII: Rëpartition of patients according to the molecules used in the medical treatment of thoracic pathologies.

Molecules	Number (n=581)	Percentage (%)
Analgesic	563	96,90
Antibiotic	456	78,48
Antihypertensive	380	65,40
Cough suppressant	354	60,92
LMWH	258	44,40
Antiplatelet agent	231	39,75
Corticoi'de	221	38,03
Antihistamine	182	31,32
NSAIDS	176	30,29
Statin	114	19,62
Anti-secretary	80	13,76

Analgesics (96.90%), antibiotics (78.48%) and antihypertensives (65.40%) were the most frequently associated medical treatments in thoracic pathology.

> **Surgical treatment**

Table XXXIII: Breakdown of patients by surgical procedure performed in thoracic surgery.

Surgical procedures	Number (n=581)	Percentage (%)
Pleural drainage	277	68,90
Pleural biopsies for mesothelioma	2	0,49
Exeresis of bronchopulmonary mass	8	1,99
Pulmonary bullectomy	3	0,74
Hydatid cyst exeresis	2	0,49
Pericardial drainage	83	20,64
Mediastinal mass examination	3	0,74
Thyroidectomy	5	1,24
Exeresis of chest wall mass	10	2,48
Diaphragmatic hernia repair	3	0,74
Mastectomy	8	1,99
Percutane hepatic drainage	3	0,74
Pneumectomy	2	0,49

Pleural and pericardial drainage were the most frequently performed procedures in thoracic surgery with a proportion of 68.90% and 20.64% respectively.

5.6.2 Vascular pathologies :

Medical treatment :

Table XXXIV: Distribution of patients according to the molecules used in the medical treatment of vascular pathologies.

Molecules	Number (n=1139)	Percentage (%)
Analgesic	1055	92,62
Antibiotic	879	77,17
NSAIDS	286	25,10

	18	1,58
Corticoid		
Antihi stamini que	199	17,47
Antihypertensive	780	68,48
Veinotonic	380	33,36
Statin	832	73,04
Antiplatelet agent	932	81,82
Antifungal	244	21,42
Anti-secretary	165	14,48
LMWH	746	65,49
VKA	312	27,39
Heparin sodium	318	27,91

Analgesics (92.62%), platelet anti-aggregants (81.82%), antibiotics (77.17%) and statins (73.04%) were the drugs most frequently used in vascular pathology.

Table XXXV: Distribution of patients according to the surgical procedures performed in vascular surgery.

Surgical procedures	Number (n=1139)	Percentage (%)
Manufacture of AVFs for hemodialysis	182	46,66
Limb amputation	95	24,35
Debridement - necrosectomy	45	11,53
Stripping vein Saphene	30	7,69
Flattening prosthetic graft for AAA	11	2,82
Aponevrotomy	10	2,56
Arterial embolectomy	6	1,53
Femoro-popliteal angioplasty	6	1,53
Implantable chamber	5	1,28
Femoropopliteal bypass	2	0,51
Exeresis of compressive lipoma	2	0,51
Flattening - resection - bypass for aneurysm	2	0,51
Temporal artery biopsies	2	0,51
Endarterectomy	1	0,25
Exeresis of popliteal cyst	1	0,25

AVF insertion for hëmodialysis (46.66%) and limb amputation (24.35%) were the main surgical procedures performed in vascular surgery.

> **Other therapies in vascular surgery**

Table XXXVI: Rëpartition of patients according to other therapeutic modes rëalisës for vascular pathology.

Other modes	Number (n=1139)	Percentage (%)
Dressing	866	76,03
Elastic restraint	137	12,02
Wearing elastic stockings	324	28,44
Limb elevation	165	14,48

Local care (76.03%) and the wearing of elastic support stockings (28.44%) were often associated with medical or surgical treatment for vascular pathology.

5.7- Evolutionary aspects

5.7.1- In thoracic surgery :

Table XXXVII: Distribution of patients according to immediate operative sequelae in thoracic surgery.

Post-operative care	Number (n=402	Percentage (%)
Simple	287	71,39
Complicated	115	28,61

The post-operative course was straightforward in 71.39% of patients.

5.7.1.1-   Breakdown by type of immediate complication:

Table XXXVIII: Rëpartition of patients according to the type of immëdiate complication in thoracic surgery.

Type of complications	Number (n=402)		Percentage (%)
Hemorrhage	9	2,23	
Dyspnea	103		25,62
Lymphoree	3	0,74	

25.62% of thoracic opërës patients had post opëratory dvspnea in thoracic surgery.

5.7.1.2-   Breakdown by late complications :

Table XXXIX: Distribution of patients according to late complications in thoracic surgery.

Complications	3 months	6 months	12 months
Chronic parietal suppuration	0,49%	0	0
Dyspnea	30,34%	13,43%	2,73%
Recurrence of effusion	3,73%	3,98%	8,95%

Dyspnea persisted in 30.34% of patients in the 3 months following the operation, and 8.95% of recurrences of effusion were observed after 12 months in thoracic surgery.

5.7.1.3-   Breakdown by hospital mortality :

Table XL: Breakdown of patients treated in hospital for thoracic surgery.

Mortality in thoracic surgery	Number (n=59)		Percentage (%)
Acute pericarditis	9		15,26
Chronic constructive pericarditis	1		1,69
Secondary pleural effusion		47	79,67
Pleural mesothelioma	1		1,69
Pneumectomy	1		1,69
TOTAL		59	100,00

5.7.2- In vascular surgery :

5.7.2.1-   Breakdown by immediate post-operative outcome

Table XLI: Distribution of patients according to immediate operative sequelae in vascular surgery.

Post-operative care	Number (n=390)	Percentage (%)
Simple	344	88,20
Complicated	46	11,80

5.7.2.2- Breakdown by type of immediate complication:

Table XLII: Rëpartition of patients according to the type of immëdiate complications in vascular surgery.

Type of complication	Number (n=390)	Percentage (%)
Arterial thrombosis	25	6,41
Hdmorrhage	14	3,58
Water lily	7	1,79

Arterial thrombosis (6.41%), riiemoiTagy (3.58%) ëwere the main complications immëdiate in vascular surgery.

Table XLIII: Rëpartition of patients according to late complications in vascular surgery.

Late complications	3 months	6 months	< 12 months
Chronic paridontal suppuration	0,76%	1,28%	0
Hematoma on AVF	1,79%	1,02%	0
AVF thrombosis	2,82%	1,28%	4,61%
False andvrism on FAV	0	0	2,82%

Late complications mainly concerned AVF for hemodialysis.

5.7.2.3- Distribution according to hospital mortality in vascular surgery:

Table XLIV: Breakdown of patients dëcëdës in hospital vascular surgery.

Mortality in vascular surgery	Number (n=43)	Percentage (%)
IRCT	9	20,93
AOMI stage 4	28	65,11
AAAR	3	6,98
Aortic dissection	3	6,98
Total	**43**	**100,00**

5.7.3- Breakdown by overall mortality in the department

Table XLV: Rëpartition of patients according to overall mortality on the ward.

Mortality	Number (N=1720)	Percentage (%)
Thoracic pathology	59	3,43
Vascular pathology	43	2,50
Total	**102**	**5,93**

Overall hospital mortality was 5.93%. Only one (1) patient died during surgery.

5.7.4- Length of stay :

Table XLVI: Rëpartition according to length of stay in intensive care.

Type of pathology	Minimum	Average	Maximum
Thoracic	< 24h	2 days	5 days
Vascular	< 24h	24 h	3 days

The average length of stay in intensive care was 2 24-hour days for thoracic surgery and vascular surgery.

Table XLVII: Rëpartition according to length of post-resuscitation hospitalisation.

Type of pathology	Minimum	Average	Maximum
Thoracic	< 24 h	5 days	
Vascular	< 24 h	3 days	14 days 8 days

In the post-resuscitation phase, the average hospital stay was 5 days for thoracic surgery and 3 days for vascular surgery.

VI. Discussion

6.1 Methodology:

A few difficulties were ëlë reported relating to the retrospective nature of the study. These concerned missing data, the archiving of files and also in the organisation of surgical activities. In fact, the Andre Festoc Centre was initially dedicated to paediatric cardiac surgery. Most of these surgical activities were carried out by foreign missionaries, which often had an impact on the management of thoracic and vascular pathologies. Some of the difficulties were related to costs and the supply of consumables.

Despite these difficulties, this work has enabled us to gain an understanding of the most common thoracic and vascular pathologies, and to identify organisational and therapeutic shortcomings in their management, in order to develop strategies and prospects for improving the quality of care.

6.2 Frequency of thoracic and vascular pathologies:

In five (5) years, 1720 patients have been seen in the department for thoracic or vascular pathology. Over the last three years, we have seen a marked increase in the number of such patients being seen. This figure seems lower than the national annual report of the Society of Thoracic and Vascular Surgery **in Japan** [36] and **Taiwan** [37]. In sub-Saharan Africa, data on the frequency of thoracic and vascular pathologies appear to be scarce. We believe that this is partly due to the scarcity and inaccessibility of specialists, but also to the fact that we are a young department with limited resources.

6.3 Epidemiological profile of specialities

6.3.1 Socio-demographic characteristics :

> **Depending on age** :

The average age of thoracic pathology patients was 44.65 years, with extremes of 2 months and 94 years. This mean age is comparable to those observed by **Souleymane. A N [38]**, **OTIOBANDA G F [39]** and **Mirande K T [40]** of 38.87, 39.07 and 34.30 years respectively. This could be explained by the youth of the African population.

In vascular pathology, the average age of patients was 54.60 years, with extremes of 3 and 123 years. This result is comparable to that of **Staniszewska. A et al [41]** who found a mean age of 67.5 years. The vascular pathologies most often dëgënëratives are the prerogative of the *elderly* subject.

> **By gender** :

In this study, women predominated in thoracic pathology rather than vascular pathology. Some authors (**Souleymane. A N [24], MIRANDE KT [40] and Staniszewska. A et al [41]** have reported a male predominance in both thoracic and vascular pathology. This predominance of women could be explained by the infectious etiology in thoracic pathologies and venous etiology in vascular pathologies, but also by the fact that many women are referred to our department due to the name of the CHU "Mother-Child".

> **By main occupation** :

All social strata are affected to varying degrees by thoracic and vascular pathologies in this study (housewives, shopkeepers, retired civil servants, schoolchildren and farmers). Thoracic and vascular diseases are generally ubiquitous.

> **Depending on origin :**

Patients came from a variety of backgrounds. The majority (93.43%) of patients were referred from the various university hospital centres (CHU) in the Bamako health district, 2.38% from reference health centres and 1.8% from regional hospitals. This could be explained by the lack of a referral service for thoracic and vascular pathologies, the quality of the technical facilities and the improved care provided by the various foreign missions.

6.3.2 Thoracic pathologies encountered :

Pleural effusions, with 293 patients, constituted the primary thoracic pathology in this study. Pleural effusion was present in 94.63% of patients. These observations have been reported by other authors with different proportions such as **Konate. F [42]** with 4.49% and **Bemba ELP [43]** with 23.11%. This variability in the frequency of pleurisy could be explained by the location of these studies. All pleurisy resistant to puncture are referred to thoracic surgery for pleural drainage.

These pleurisies may progress to pyothorax. We recorded 4.72% pyothorax. This result is comparable to the 1.95% reported by **Guindo. I O [45]** in 2013 at the "G" point university hospital. In this ëtude we reported two cases of post traumatic he'mothorax. I . hemothorax is most often secondary to closed trauma with a variable frequency between 25.2 - 32% according to some West African studies [46,47].

With 22.3%, pericardial spasm was the second most frequent thoracic pathology in this study. This frequency is comparable to the 1.78% reported by **DIOP. S [48]** in 2022 in a hospital in Mali, the 2.6% reported by **HAIDARA O T [49]** and the 0.21% reported by KONE B [50]. This variability of results could be explained by the fact that we are a reference department for cardiac surgery in the country and in the sub-region.

With 34 patients, broncho-pleural masses constituted the 3eme thoracic pathology in this study. Only 6.20% benefited from a histological diagnosis because of the advanced stage. Thoracic trauma was observed in 28 patients. These thoracic injuries accounted for 4.30% of thoracic surgery. This result is comparable to those of **Fadima Tall [52]** with 1.02% and **Coulibaly. S [53]** with 0.87%.

Plunging goitres were the most common pathology at the upper border of the thorax, with 14 patients treated, representing 2.40% of all thoracic surgery cases. The rate of plunging goitres in thyroid surgery varies in the literature from 2% to 30% **[54, 55]**.

In our study, twelve (12) patients had a parestinal mass, 25% of which was located in the suprasternal and subclavicular regions. **El Hachimi. K et al [56]** reported 5.3% supraclavicular masses.

Hiatal hernia is a less common lower thoracic border disease. We enrolled 11 patients, three (3) of whom underwent conventional surgery.

We collected data on 8 patients with advanced pulmonary emphysema. Three patients underwent successful surgery for giant emphysema bullae.

Six (6) patients had a mediastinal mass. These were generally malignant tumours as reported in the literature [57] with signs of compression (chest pain, dyspnSe, cough) [58].

6.3.3- Vascular pathologies encountered :

With 399 patients coШgës, përiphëric arteriopathies of the limbs represented the first vascular pathology managed in the department. The majority of these were atheromatous degenerative arteriopathy. These patients most often consulted at an advanced stage (Leriche and Fontaine stage 4) with a high risk of amputation.

The therapeutic management of chronic end-stage renal failure involves hemodialysis. This therapeutic strategy requires the creation of a high-quality vascular approach. Out of 262 patients with renal failure referred to the department, an arteriovenous fistula (AVF) was created in 182 patients. This result is comparable to the 112 patients who benefited from AVF in the study conducted by **Dieng. P A et al [60]** in Dakar.

DVT, with 121 patients managed, was the third most common vascular pathology in this study. It was located in the lower limbs in 91.73% of patients. **Haounou. F et al [61]** reported a rate of 51.3%.

Venous insufficiency of the lower limbs was diagnosed in 121 patients, representing 10.6% of vascular pathologies. Chronic venous insufficiency accounted for 60.33%. **Konin. C et al [63]** reported a prevalence of 60.4% of chronic venous insufficiency of the lower limbs. Chronic venous disease of the lower limbs is a major cause of morbidity and reduced quality of life, affecting up to 25% of western populations **[62]**. All patients diagnosed with CVI have benefited from the prescription of lifestyle hygiene measures and elastic venous compression. CVI appears to be common in the black African population. CVL of the lower limbs most often progresses to the appearance of varicose veins. We collected 54 patients with varicose veins of the lower limbs. Varicose disease affects one third of the French population [64].

Aneurysmal disease, with 48 patients, represented 4.21% of vascular pathologies. Arterial aneurysm affects 7 to 8% of people aged over 65 in the West and is the 12th leading cause of death in these countries **[65, 66]**. In sub-Saharan Africa, arterial aneurysm is uncommon, and is probably poorly evaluated, but this is related to the scarcity of vascular surgeons [67]. Aneurysm of the subrenal abdominal aorta (AAASR) remains the most frequent location, accounting for 90% [68]. We operated on 11 patients, i.e. 23% of aneurysms.

Other përiphëric aneurysms (internal iliac, deep fëmoral, internal carotid) have been opërë with success.

Forty-one (41) patients consulted for lymphaemia, i.e. 3.59%. It was a primary ivinplicL'deme in 87,80% localisës to the pelvic limbs and secondaries in 12,20% to the thoracic limbs consëcutifs to the surgical cure of breast cancer. **SANOGO. A M [69]** reported 89.1% ivmplicL'deme of the lower limbs.

As in the ëstudies by **Vertilus. B et al [70] and HOLF** et al [71], about ten patients were managed for traumatic compartment syndrome.

Aortic dissection is a life-threatening vascular emergency. In this study, 10 patients were treated for arterial dissection. Intensive care medical treatment was systematic given the inadequacy of the technical platform.

According to **Compton C [72]**, major trauma is responsible for 3% of vascular injuries. In this study, 7 patients were treated for vascular trauma.

The implantation of central catheters for chemotherapy is a cross-disciplinary activity (intensive care unit, urologist, gynaecologist, surgeon). Five (5) patients benefited from implantation of an implantable catheter chamber.

Vascular malformations are generally rare. They may be venous, arterial or arteriovenous (AVM), consisting of multiple high-flow shunts **[79]**. Surgery is mainly reserved for progressive or complicated forms (stages II to IV). Four (4) patients were treated for arteriovenous malformation.

6.4 - Clinical aspects :

6.4.1- Risk factors and/or co-morbidities :

In thoracic pathology, the risk factors or comorbidities are well known. These are hypertension, diabetes, smoking, tuberculosis and neoplasia, which were observed in different proportions in this study.

In vascular pathology, age, hypertension, diabetes, smoking, kidney disease and heart disease were the main risk factors for vascular disease. Other factors such as previous stroke and neoplasia were present in some patients.

6.4.2 Functional signs :

6.4.2.1 Thoracic diseases :

Chest pain (87.43%), dyspnoea (75.90%) and cough (18.58%) were the main symptoms on admission to thoracic surgery. The intensity of these signs was most often related to the patient's condition and antecedents, but also to the stage at which the disease was evolving.

A pleural effusion syndrome, in particular dullness, reduced vesicular murmur and reduced vocal vibration, was present in the majority of patients.

6.4.2.2 Vascular pathologies :

Limb pain (88.05%), reduced walking range (less than 150 m) (41.27%) and intermittent arterial claudication (23.88%) were the main symptoms observed in vascular pathology. This result could be explained by the high frequency of peripheral degenerative arteriopathy.

Limb tumefaction (47.41%), absence of pulse (40.82%) and cyanosis (26.07%) were the major signs observed in vascular pathology. These signs are most often seen in peripheral arteriopathy and chronic venous insufficiency.

6.5 Additional examinations

6.5.1- Radiological :

In thoracic pathology, imaging is of the utmost importance and is guided by the clinic, forming the basis of the diagnostic work-up. Chest radiography (85.71%) remains the examination of first choice. Thoracic CT (28.05%) is indispensable for the therapeutic management of thoracic pathologies, providing a more accurate diagnosis of lesions.

In vascular pathology, in addition to clinical symptoms, radiological examinations are necessary for diagnosis. Arterial and venous Doppler ultrasound of the limbs (61.36%) and angioscanner (14.22%) were the main imaging examinations carried out for the diagnosis of vascular pathologies. In fact, angioscanner is an essential morphological and hemodynamic examination that is indispensable for therapeutic management in vascular pathology.

Thoracic and vascular surgery is major surgery. Whatever the pathology, it is necessary to carry out an assessment of the patient's condition and also a cardiac assessment to minimise the risks associated with surgery. Cardiac ultrasound (79.17%) and ECG (71.08%) were the main examinations carried out for this cardiac assessment.

6.5.2 Biological :

Biological tests are used to assess the impact of these pathologies on the various organs. CBC (48.77%), creatinineemia (40.34%), blood urea (29.76%), CRP (43.95%), blood ionogram (27.15%) and transaminases (38.02%) constituted the initial biological work-up carried out in thoracic and vascular pathology. Rhesus grouping, PT and APTT were used to complete the preoperative work-up. Histological examination of all surgical specimens was systematic.

In the search for specific etiologies in certain areas, other complementary examinations were carried out. Gen Xpert (195 patients) and ECBC (174 patients) were performed systematically for pleuropericardial effusions. Hepatitis B serology (168 patients), HCV serology (165 patients) and HIV serology (165 patients) were performed depending on the patient's condition.

6.6 - Therapeutic aspects :

6.6.1 Medical

Whatever the thoracic or vascular pathology, mëdico-chirurgical treatment is used. In thoracic pathology, this is most often a combination of analgesics, antibiotics, corticoids and, in particular, anti-tuberculosis drugs. This medical treatment most often accompanies the surgical treatment.

In vascular pathology, antiplatelet agents, statins, ACE inhibitors, analgesics, sometimes antibiotics, venotonics and vasodilators are the most frequently used molecules.

Other non-medicinal therapeutic strategies such as oxygen therapy, locoregional care or dressings and bandaging can provide relief.

6.6.2 Surgical :

Surgical treatment depended on the indication, the technical resources available and the patient's consent.

In thoracic pathology, 402 surgical procedures were carried out, representing 50.75% of the department's surgical activity. Pleural drainage (68.90%), xiphoid pericardial drainage (20.64%) and removal of masses (mediastinal, parietal or hydatid cysts) (5.21%) were the main procedures performed in thoracic surgery.

The main procedures performed in vascular surgery were the creation of arteriovenous fistulas for hemodialysis (46.66%), major limb amputations (24.35%) and stripping of the saphenous veins. Given the high frequency of degenerative arterial disease, bypass surgery or other revascularisation procedures should predominate in vascular surgery. We believe that lack of knowledge of vascular pathologies, delays in consultation, poverty, inaccessibility to the few specialists and inadequate technical facilities could explain these results.

6.7 Evolution :

6.7.1 Morbidity :

I The clinical and paraclinical evolution ëwas generally favourable in the majority of our patients.

In thoracic surgery, 71.39% of patients had an uncomplicated post-operative course. The immediate morbidity rate was 28.61%. These were essentially persistent dyspnea (89.57%) and intraoperative haemorrhage (7.83%). Medium- and long-term post-operative follow-up was marked by recurrence of the effusion in 16 patients.

In vascular surgery, postoperative revolution was simple in 88.20% of cases. Immediate complications were dominated by arterial thrombosis (54.34%), bleeding (24.44%) and lymphorrhage (15.22%). The morbidity rate was 11.80%. Medium- and long-term complications were all related to AVF for hemodialysis.

These complications are more common in thoracic surgery than in vascular surgery.

6.7.2 Mortality :

Overall hospital mortality was 5.93%. Only one (1) patient died peroperatively. Mortality in thoracic surgery was 10% and 3.7% in vascular surgery.

This mortality rate could be explained by the fact that a greater number of patients are referred by oncology, medicine and cardiology departments. These patients are usually weakened by the underlying disease, with pleural or pericardial effusions of neoplastic origin, sometimes on a background of congestive heart failure, HIV or tuberculosis.

Conclusion

Thoracic and cardiovascular surgery has been a mëdico-surgical discipline exercëe for dëcennies in Mali but a young activity at the CHU Mëre Enfant "le Luxembourg".

I. At the Andre FESTOC centre, thoracic pathology was less frequently treated than vascular pathology. Thoracic patients were younger than vascular patients. Housewives were predominant in this study. The majority of patients were referred by the CHUs or CSREFs of the Bamako district.

The main risk factors and/or comorbidities in thoracic surgery were hypertension, diabetes, smoking, pulmonary tuberculosis and neoplasia. In vascular surgery, other pathologies such as age, nephropathy and heart disease were associated.

Clinical symptomatology was dominated in thoracic pathology by chest pain, dyspnoea and cough. In vascular pathology, these were mainly pain, intermittent arterial claudication and a decrease in walking pace to less than 150m.

The dii'i erent pathologies frequently encountered in thoracic pathology were pleuropericardial effusions, parietal or mediastinal masses or bronchopulmonary masses. The dominant vascular pathologies were degenerative peripheral arteriopathies, deep vein thrombosis, veno-lymphatic insufficiency, varicose veins and some vascular malformations.

Surgery has made an important therapeutic contribution. The most common surgical procedures performed in thoracic surgery were pleural or pericardial drainage, exeresis-biopsy of certain parietal or bronchopulmonary masses, thyroidectomy for plunging goitre, and often mastectomy for breast cancer. In vascular surgery, the most common surgical procedures were the creation of an AVF for hemodialysis, limb amputation, stripping for varicose veins, and the cure of arterial aneurysms.

The morbidity-mortality rate remains acceptable in the management of these pathologies in our department.

If we are to improve our results, we need to run a campaign to raise awareness of thoracic and vascular diseases so that patients can be consulted at an early stage, train paramedical staff and strengthen the technical platform by making minimally invasive techniques (thoracoscopy and endovascular surgery) more widely available.

Recommendations

At the end of this work we recommend :

To the general public:

> Join 1 Assurance Maladie Obligatoire (compulsory health insurance) to help with the cost of healthcare.

> Consult your doctor as soon as you notice any serious chest or vascular symptoms.

> Avoid certain situations or risk factors for chest and vascular disease.

> Encouraging all types of sport.

Social and health care staff :

> Early treatment of patients suffering from thoracic and/or vascular pathology.

> Good collaboration between different specialities to improve the quality of care in hospitals.

To the political and administrative authorities:

> Popularise public awareness campaigns on non-communicable diseases, in particular thoracic and cardiovascular pathologies.

> Providing initial and continuing training for spëcialists in thoracic and vascular surgery.

> Subsidising the medical and surgical management of thoracic and vascular pathologies.

> Create other centres of excellence for the management of thoracic and vascular pathologies.

> Strengthen the technical facilities of hospitals, especially in terms of less invasive techniques, to improve the quality of care.

REFERENCES

[1] Ba. M S. Thoracic and cardiovascular surgery in a developing country (review of activity at Dakar University Hospital). These medecine. 1ᵉ February 1997. 147. P27-44

[2] SMITH J A., MULLERWORTH M H., WESTLAKE G W., TATOULIS J.Empyema thoraces: a 14 years experiences in a teaching center.Ann thoracic surg 1991; 51:P39- 42.

[3] Dr Maurice Perol, Departement Prevention Cancer Environnement, Centre Leon Berard pneumologue cancerologue, Centre Leon Berard, Lyon. Updated on 20 July 2023.

[4] Nganmeni Ignace. THORACIC SURGICAL PATHOLOGIES IN THE SURGICAL DEPARTMENT A OF THE HOPITAL DU POINT-G: REVIEW OF CASES. Faculte de Medecine, de Pharmacie et d'Odonto-Stomatologie. 2006. 121. P22-24

[5] Dieng. P A, Ciss. G, Ba. P S, Ndiaye. A, Fall. M B. Gaye. M, Diatta. S Kane. O, Beye. S A. Diarra. O, Diouf. B, Ndiaye. M. Results of arteriovenous fistulas for chronic hemodialysis in Dakar. Service de chirurgie thoracique et cardiovasculaire de CHU de FANN. African Journal of Surgery 2010; 1(1): 74-77.

[6] Konin. C et al. Chronic venous insufficiency in a black African population: epidemiological and therapeutic aspects and determining factors. Journal of Vascular Diseases. Volume 40, issue 2, march 2015 Page 123.

[7] Haounou. F, Binjilali. L, Zahlane. M, Essaadouni. L. venous thromboenbolic disease in internal medicine: a descriptive study of 157 hospitalised patients. La revue de la medecine interne, volume 37 , Supplement 2 decembre 2016, pages A148-A149.

[8] James Didier L., Abdoulaye MB. Bako H. Ide K., Saidou A., Ide G., Hama Y., Sani Rabiou. Chaibou MS, Daddy H. Adakal O. Sidibe T. Ouaissi M. Harouna Y. Abarchi H. Sani R. Prise En Charge Des Anevrismes Arteriels Dans Un Centre Africain Non Specialisee. European Scientific Journal January 2018 edition Vol.14, No.3 ISSN: 1857 - 7881 (Print) e - ISSN 1857- 7431.

[9] Nganmeni Ignace. THORACIC SURGICAL PATHOLOGIES IN THE SURGICAL DEPARTMENT A OF THE HOPITAL DU POINT-G: REVIEW OF CASES. Faculte de Medecine, de Pharmacie et d'Odonto-Stomatologie. 2006.

[10] Guindo. I O.Aspects epidemiologiques, evolutifs et therapeutiques des pleuresies purulentes au service de pneumo-phtisiologie du CHU Point G. faculte de medecine et odonto-stomatologie. 2013.

[11] PAUL LECENE. Histoire de la chirurgie, Flammarion, 1923, PARIS.

[12] ROBERT B. WAGNER M D. and BENJAMIN SLIVKO M D. highlights of the history of nonpenetrating chest trauma, surgical clinics of the north amerca, 1989, 69, 1-12.

[13] DIOP HENRITTE CECILE AMINATA. Aspects chirurgicaux du traitement de la tuberculose pleuropulmonaire, thesis med, Dakar 1993, N° 59.

[14] DIEYE OUSMANE. Prise en charge des traumatismes vasculaires des membres, these de medecine, DAKAR 1994, N° 17.

[15] GONTARSKI J J. certificate of need : cardiac diagnostic, facilities and cardiac surgery centers, New Jersey administrativr CODE NJAC, 1986, 8; 33E.

[16] ANTHONY R C. DOBELL M D. Rival trailblazers: the origins of successful closed valvular surgery, the annals of thoracic surgery, 1996, 61 7506 754.

[17] Hermes C. GRILLO. Congenital lesions neoplasms and injuries of the trachea. Gibbon's surgery of the chest (fourth edition). W B. SAUNDERS Philadelphia 1983. 1 . 244-245.

[18] Alain the warrior. New anatomy files - PECM. Thorax 2ᵉᵐᵉ edution.

[19] Richard L. Drake, A. Wayne Vogl, Adam W. M. Mitchell. Anatomie pour les etudiants 3ᵉᵐᵉ French edition coordinated by Fabrice Duparc and jacques Duparc

[20] Richard W. Light, MD, Vanderbilt University Medical Center review/revision complete Jan. 2021

[21] CHUV Department of Cardiology Rue du Bugnon 46 CH-1011 Lausanne, Vaud, Switzerland. 31/01/2023. N° 23

[22] Geneva University Hospitals. Endocrine surgery. 04/05/2021. N°17

[23] Jacquelline Rossant-Lumbroso, Lyonel Rossant. Les arteriopathies. Doctissimo on 03.07. 2019.

[24] F. Becker. Arteriopathies of the upper limb, Revue Medicale Suisse 2007; volume 3. 31999.

[25] Lachomette, Konecna, macheda. Arterial fistula. Arterial and venous surgery. 24.07.2020.

[26] G. Franco. J. Marzelle. Explorations de la fistule arterioveineuse. 07/10/2019. [18-024-Q- 10] - Doi: 10.1016/S1762-0945(19)64215-4.

[27] Vidal. Les medicaments de la thrombose veineuse. 01 July 2022.

[28] Federation francaise de cardiologie. Venous insufficiency: situations at risk Publication date: 8 October 2016 - Amended on 21 May 2021 -

[29] Danielle Campagne, MD. compartment syndrome. University of california, San Francisco. Medical examination dec. 2022.

[30] BOURGUIGNON T. Le drainage pleural, Unite de Chirurgie Thoracique - CHU de Tours, 2007.

[31] Nganmeni I, Surgical thoracic pathologies in the surgical service A of the hopital du point-G: case review. 2006.

[32] LA Mine. Hospital and prehospital emergency medicine. Gestes thoraciques d'exception en medecine d'urgence.7 novembre 2015

[33] Alain Branchereau, Pierre-Edouard Magan, Eugenio Rosset. Voies D'abord des Vaisseaux. 1995.

[34] Ricco. J.B, Sessa.C. approaches to the abdominal aorta and iliac arteries. EMC 43- techniques chirurgicales- chirurgie vasculaire, 43-034-A.2010

[35] Madioke Mahamadou DIAWARA. Diagnostic aspects of hemothorax secondary to firm trauma of the thorax in the Thoracic Surgery Department of the Mali Hospital. 15 / 01 / 2022.

[36] Shunsuke. Endo et al. Thoracic and cardiovascular surgery in Japan in 2016. General Thoracic and cardiovascular surgery 67, 377-477 (2019).

[37] Xing. Gao and Yin-Kai. Chao. Thoracic surgery in Taiwan. Journal of thoracic disease 2022 Jul; 14(7): 2712-2720.

[38] Souleymane. A N, thoracic surgery: evaluation of anaesthesiological management at the CHU du point G. faculte de medecine et odontostomatolgie 26/12 /2013.

[39] Otiobanda G.F., Mahougou-Guimbi K.C., Bodzongo D. Anaesthesia for thoracic surgery at Brazzaville University Hospital. Congres de la societe d'anesthesie Reanimation d'Afrique Noire Francophone. Dakar, November 2011, C49, p26

[40] Komguem Tagne Mirande. Selective intubation in thoracic surgery at Point G Hospital. Our first experience. These medecine, Bamako 06M33.

[41] Staniszewska. A, Gimzewska. M, Onida. S, Voie. T, and Dqvies A H. limb arterial interventions in England. Ann R Coll Surg Engl. 20121 May ; 103(5) : 360 - 366.

[42] Konate. F. epidemio-clinical and etiological aspects of pleurisy with clear liquid of the old subject in the pneumo-phtisiology service of the university hospital of the pointG. Faculte de medecine et odonto-stomatologie de Bamako. 2020.

[43] Bemba ELP, Ossale abacka KB, Koumeka PP, Okemba okombi FH, Bopaka RG, Mboussa J. Profil des affections respiratoires du sujet age au service de pneumologie du chu de Brazzaville. Annales de l'Universite Marien NgOUABI 2018;18(1):19-27.

[44] Adambounou AS, Adjoh KS, Hamadou BB,Fiogbe A A0, Aziagbe KA, Efalou PJ, Gbadamassi G, Boukari M, Kombate D, Akpo K. Etiologies of pleurisy in the elderly in Togo. European Scientific Journal October 2015;11(30):1857-7881.

[45] Guindo. I O.Aspects epidemiologiques, evolutifs et therapeutiques des pleuresies purulentes au service de pneumo-phtisiologie du CHU Point G. faculte de medecine et odonto-stomatologie. 2013.

[46] VIVIEN B, RIOU B. Traumatismes thoraciques graves : Strategie diagnostique et thera peutique. EMC (Elvier Mason SAS). : 36-725-C-20 (2003) 27.

[47] NIKIEMA A. Post-traumatic hemothorax at the CHU-YO: epidemiological, clinical, para-clinical, therapeutic and evolutionary aspects. A propos de 52 cas colliges. These de medecine, Oua gadougou. 2012, 94p

[48] Diop. S, Prise en charge chirurgicale des pericardites dans le service de chirurgie thoracique de l'hopital du Mali. Faculte de medecine et d'odonto-stomatologie. 2022.

[49] Haidara OT. Diagnosis etiologique et évolution des pericardites dans les services de cardiologie des CHU du Point "G" et Gabriel TOURE d'Avril 2005 a Decembre 2006. These de medecine, CHU Point G de Bamako, 2008; p41-65.

[50] Kone B. Anatomopathological diagnosis of Pericarditis at the CHU du Point G de Bamako. Oct. 2017. These de medecine,CHU Point G Bamak, 2017;p1-44. Available at: http://www.keneya.net/fmpos/theses/2017/med/pdf/17M185.pdf

[51] Yena S, Togo S, Ouattara M et al. Chronic pericarditis: indications and surgical results of 31 cases observed in Bamako. Afrique Thorax Creur et Vaisseaux. 2011;- 1(2):24-29.

[52] Tall F. Etude epidemiologique, clinique et therapeutique des traumatismes thoraciques au service d'accueil des urgences du CHU Gabriel TOURE. These de medecine. Bamako, 2010, n 88,78P.

[53] Coulibaly. S. Urgences traumatiques fermes du thorax au SAU de L'HDM : interet l'imagerie medicale dans la prise en charge. Faculte de medecine et d'odonto-stomatologie de Bamako. 2021.

[54] White ML, Doherty GM, Gauger PG. Evidence-based surgical management of substernal goiter. World J Surg 2008;32: 1285-300.

[55] Cichon S, Anielski R, Konturek A,Baczynski M, Uchon W, Orlicki B. Surgicalmanagement of mediastinal goiter: risk factor for sternotomy. Langenbecks Arch Surg 2008;393:751-7.

[56] El Hachimi. K et Al. Thoracic parietal masses. Revue des maladies respiratpires. Volume 32, Supplement, january 2015, Page A119.

[57] Gonzalez. M et al. What should be done about an anterior mediastinal mass in adults? Management of anterior mediastinal masses in adults. Revue des maladies respiratoires. Volume 29, number 2, February 2012, pages 138 -148.

[58] Duwe. BV et al. Tumours of the mediastinum. Chest 2005

[59] Niang B. limb amputation for arteriopathy: Etude de l'evolution des patients au service de chirurgie thoracique et cardiovasculaire du CHU de FANN A PROPOS DE 37 CASES. Cheikh Anta Diop University, Dakar, 2016.

[60] Nganmeni I, Surgical thoracic pathologies in the surgical department A of the hopital du point-G: case review. 2006.

[61] Haounou. F, Binjilali. L, Zahlane. M, Essaadouni. L. venous thromboenbolic disease in internal medicine: a descriptive study of 157 hospitalised patients. La revue de la medecine interne, volume 37 , Supplement 2 decembre 2016, pages A148-A149.

[62] Xing. Gao and Yin-Kai. Chao. Thoracic surgery in Taiwan. Journal of thoracic disease 2022 Jul; 14(7): 2712-2720.

[63] Konin. C et al. Chronic venous insufficiency in a black African population: epidemiological and therapeutic aspects and determining factors. Journal of Vascular Diseases. Volume 40, issue 2, march 2015 Page 123.

[64] Mathieu Josnin, Nicolas Neaume. Review of endovenous treatments for varicose veins of the lower limbs. Sang thrombose vaisseaux 2018, 30, numéroero 3 : 113 - 23.

[65] Ricco JB, Regnault de la Mothe G. Surgery of arterial aneurysms of the limbs. Encycl Med Chir , Techniques chirurgicales - Chirurgie vasculaire 43-028-A. 2011 ; 21p.

[66] Deglise S, Dubuis C, Francois S et al. Diagnostic and therapeutic management of thoracic and/or abdominal aortic aneurysms.Forum Med Suisse.2013 ;13(37) :719-724.

[67] James Didier L., Abdoulaye MB. Bako H. Ide K., Saidou A., Ide G., Hama Y., Sani Rabiou. Chaibou MS, Daddy H. Adakal O. Sidibe T. Ouaissi M. Harouna Y. Abarchi H. Sani R. Prise En Charge Des Anevrismes Arteriels Dans Un Centre Africain Non Specialisee. European Scientific Journal January 2018 edition Vol.14, No.3 ISSN: 1857 - 7881 (Print) e - ISSN 1857- 7431.

[68] Baleato S, Bierry G, Garcia-Figueiras R. Anevrismes arteriels ; revue des differents territoires. Journees francaises de radiologie paris. 2008 oct: 24-28.

[69] SANOGO. A M. Epidemiological and clinical aspects of lymphoedema in the dermatology

department of the Gabriel Toure University Hospital in Bamako. Faculty of Medicine and Odonto-Stomatology. 2013

[70] B. Vertilus. Acute compartment syndrome of the limbs.INFO-CHIR:La Revue Haitienne de Chirurgie et d'Anesthesiologie Vol. 3 No. 15 Decembre 2014.

[71] [40] Hoff et al: East Practice Management Guidelines Work Group: Update to Practice Management Guidelines for Prophylactic Antibiotic Use in Open Fractures. The Journal of trauma Injury,Infection, and Critical Care - Volume 70, Number 3, March 2011.

[72] Comptom C, Rhee R. Peripheral vascular trauma. Perspect Vasc Surg Endovasc Ther 2005; 17 (4): 297-307.

[73] Ouedraogo. S , Zida. M , Tall. M, Troare S S. Results of surgical treatment of popliteal cysts in Burkina Faso. Vol. 38, numero 1 et 2 - Javier-decembre 2015, science et tchnique, sciences de la sante.

[74] Hacoubi. H, Abidallah. Haddiya. I. Giant lipomas of the limbs (about two cases and review of the literature). Rev Maroc chir orthop traumato 2011 ; 44 : 51 - 54.

[75] Crib GL; Cool WP, Ford D J, Mangham DC. Giant lipomatous tumours of the hand and forearm. J Hand surg 2005; 30B:509-12.

[76] Terzioglu. A, tuncali D, Yuksel A, Bingul F, Aslan G. Giant lipomas : a series of 12 consecutive caces and a giant liposarcoma of the thigh. Dermatol surg 2004 ; 30 : 463- 7.

[77] M. Wassef. Vascular tumours pseudo-tumours. Arterioveinous malformation. Ann Pathol 2011; 31:292-6.

[78] Hacoubi. H, Abidallah. Haddiya. I. Giant lipomas of the limbs (about two cases and review of the literature). Rev Maroc chir orthop traumato 2011 ; 44 : 51 - 54.

[79] Vanwijcka R. degardin-capon N. les malformations arterioveineues : aspects cliniques et evolution. Ann Chir Plast Esthet 2006; 51: 440-6.

[80] Casnova D. Bardot J. Bartoli J-M. Magalon G. Surgical treatment of arteriovenous malformations. Ann Chir Plast Esthet 2006 ;51 : 456-70.

Iconographies :

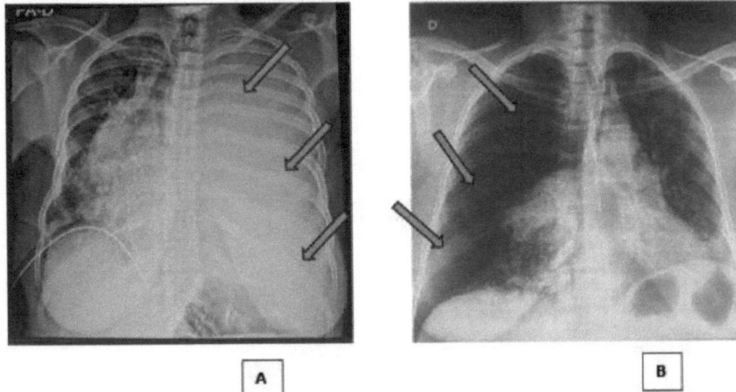

Figure 41: A. Severe left pleurisy, **B.** Right pneumothorax (Andre FESTOC Centre, CHU-ME Bamako).

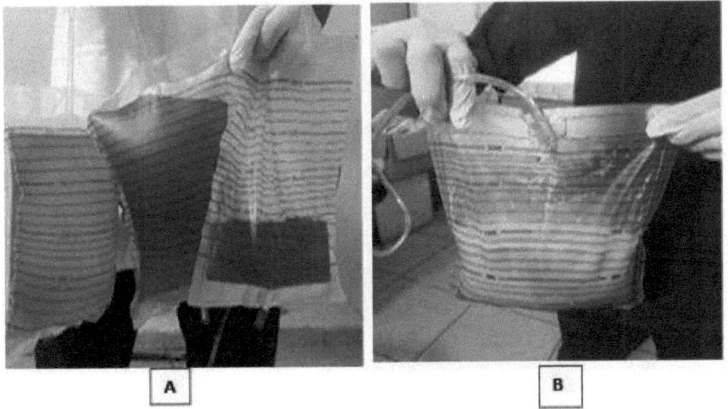

Figure 42: A. Chest drainage yielding 4500 ml of citrine yellow liquid, **B.** Chest drainage yielding 900 ml of frank pus (Andre FESTOC Centre, CHU-ME, Bamako).

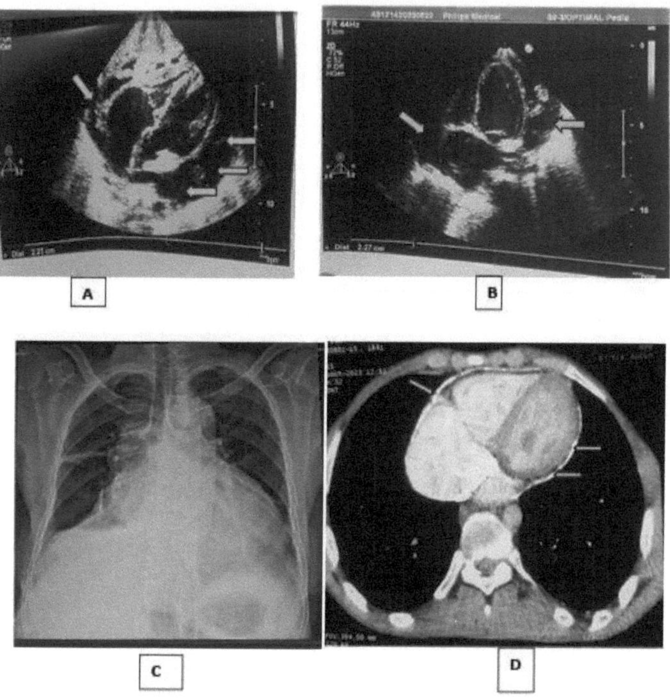

Figure 43: A, B. TTE showing large circumferential pericardial effusion, **C.** Front chest X-ray showing pleuropericardial effusion. **D.** Thoracic angioscanner showing chronic constructive pericarditis (Andre FESTOC Centre, CHU-ME, Bamako).

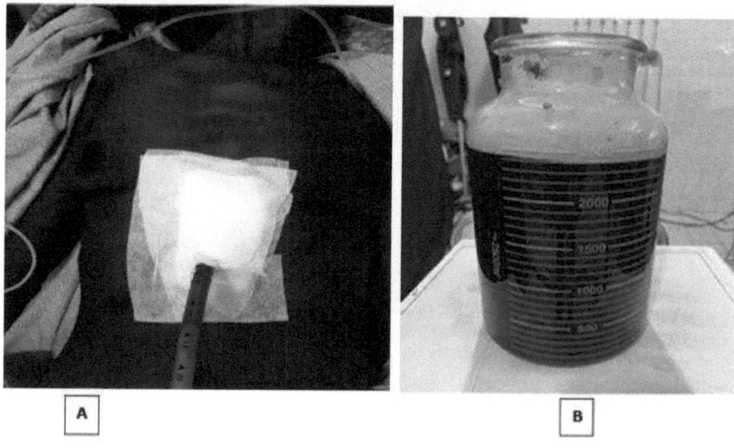

Figure 44: A. Percutaneous pericardial drainage site in an adult, **B.** Pericardial drainage returning 2500 ml of serum fluid (Andre FESTOC Centre, CHU-ME, Bamako).

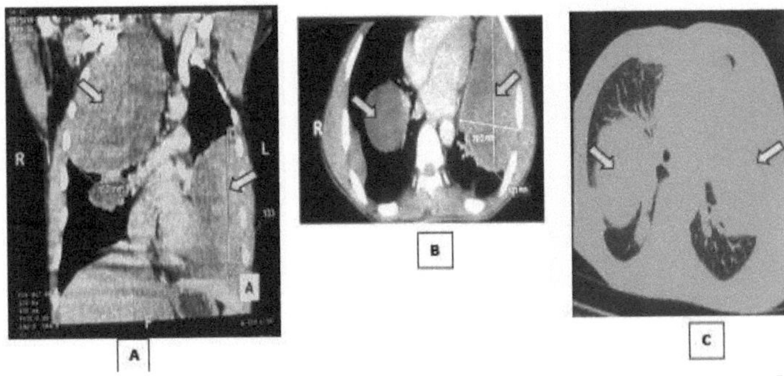

Figure 45: A,B,C. Bilateral bronchopulmonary mass. (Andre FESTOC Centre, CHU-ME, Bamako).

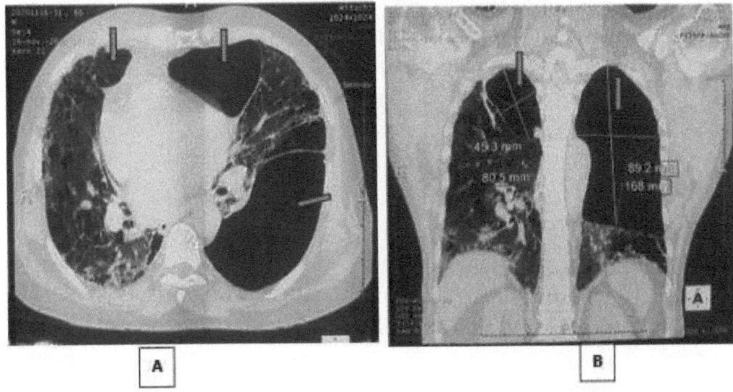

Figure 46: **A,B.** Thoracic CT scan objectiva bilateral pulmonary emphysema bullae. (Andre FESTOC Centre, CHU-ME Bamako).

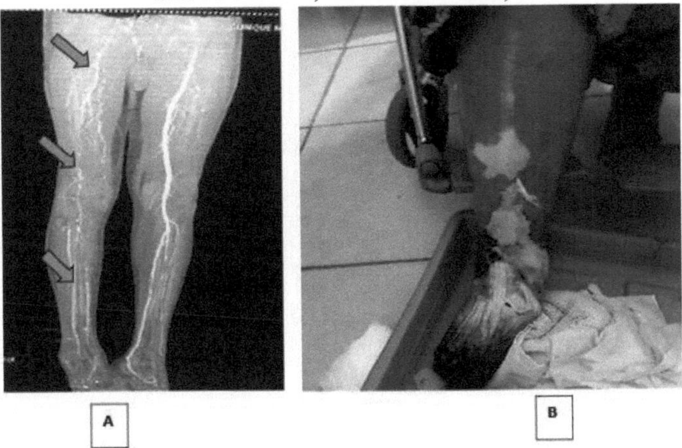

Figure 47: **A.** Angioscan of the IM showing arteriopathy more marked on the right, **B.** Mixed gangrene of the MID (Andre FESTOC Centre, CHU-ME, Bamako).

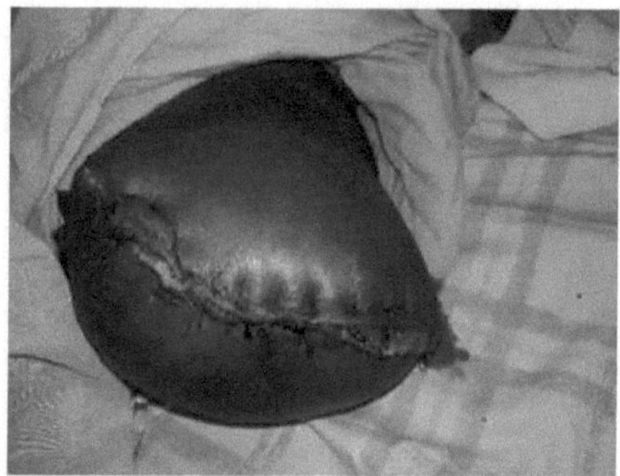

Figure 48: Right thigh amputation stump (Andre FESTOC Centre, CHU-ME, Bamako).

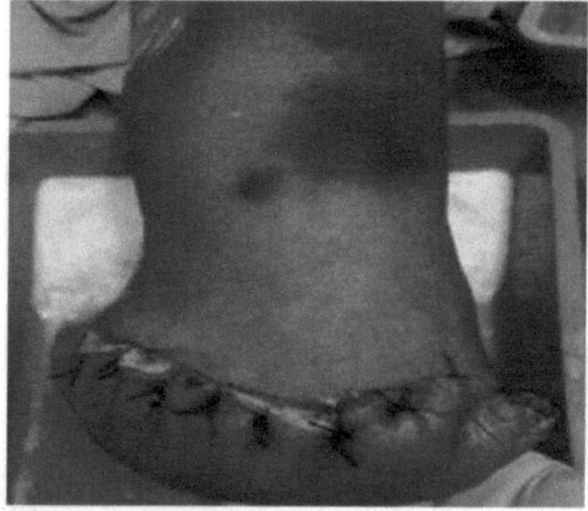

Figure 49: Left leg amputation stump (Andre FESTOC Centre, CHU-ME, Bamako).

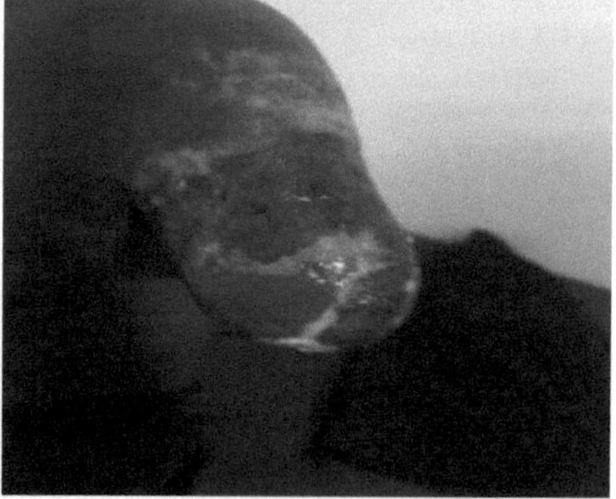

Figure 50: Left arm amputation stump in a child. (Andre FESTOC Centre, CHU-ME, Bamako).

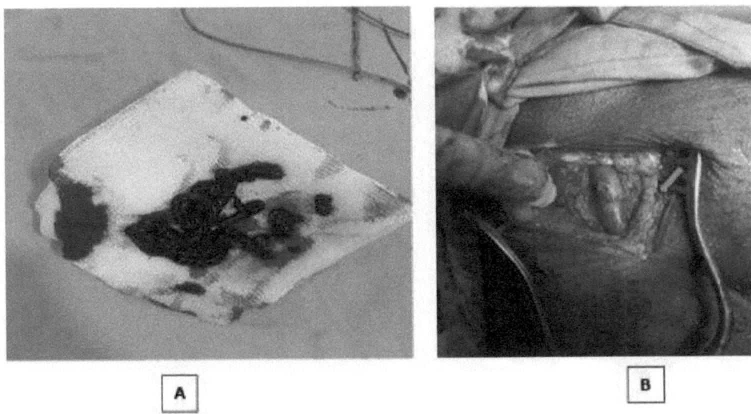

Figure 51: A. Embolectomy specimen; **B.** Arteriotomy of the right femoral tripod post embolectomy. (Andre FESTOC Centre, CHU-ME, Bamako).

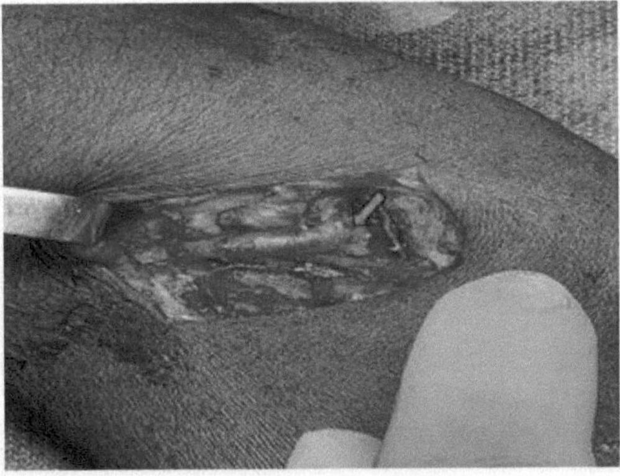

Figure 52: Left humerocephalic anastomosis (Andre FESTOC Centre, CHU-ME, Bamako).

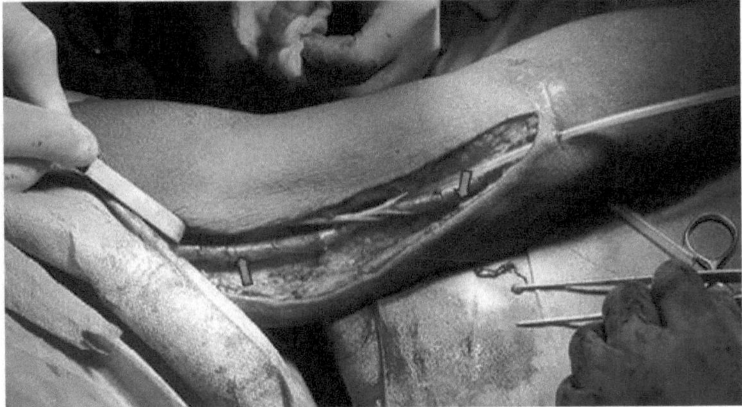

Figure 53: Superficialization of the right basilic vein following humeral-basilic anastomosis (Andre FESTOC Centre, CHU-ME, Bamako).

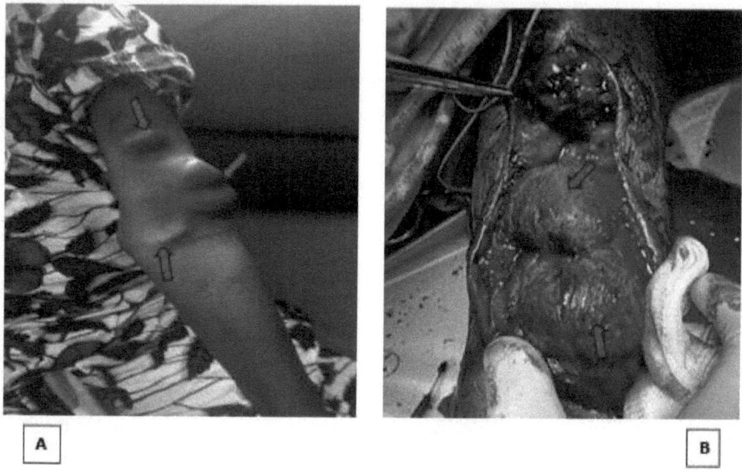

Figure 54: A. False aneurysm on AVF **B.** Demonstration of false aneurysm. (André FESTOC Centre, CHU-ME of Bamako).

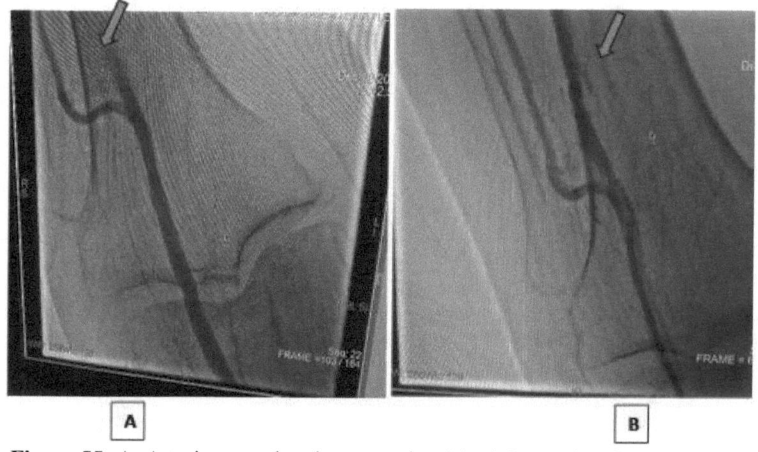

Figure 55: A. Arteriogram showing stenosis of the left anterior tibial artery, **B.** Arteriography showing repermeabilisation of the same tibial artery following angioplasty (Centre André FESTOC CHU-ME, Bamako).

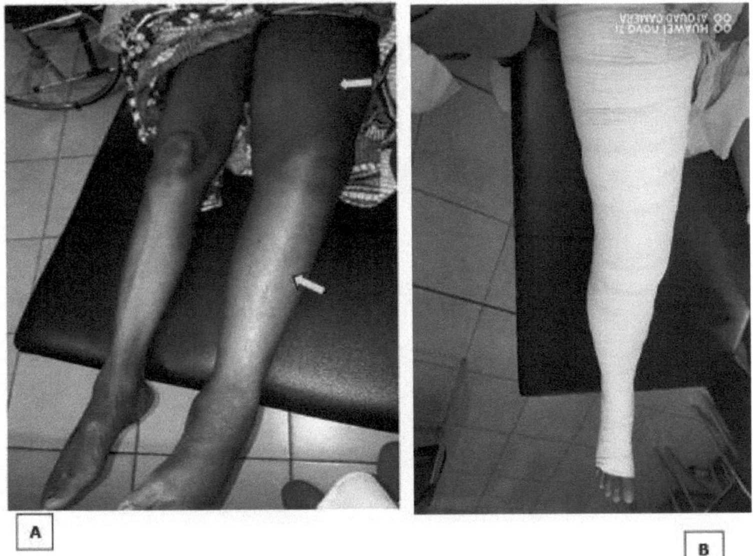

Figure 56: A. DVT of the MIG, **B.** Post DVT compression with elastic band. (Andre FESTOC Centre, CHU-ME, Bamako).

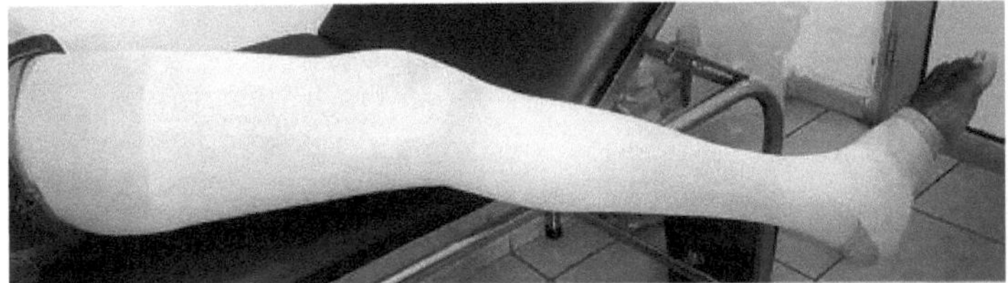

Figure 57: Support stockings for CVI. (Andre FESTOC Centre, CHU-ME, Bamako).

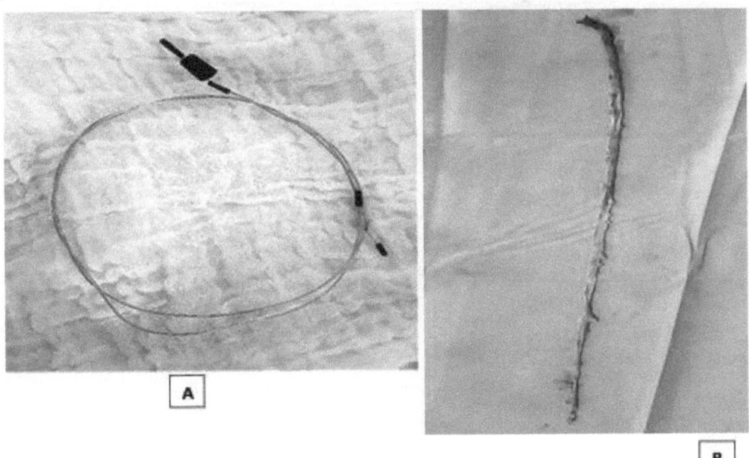

Figure 58: A. Stripper, **B.** Eveinage by stripping the right great saphenous vein (Andre

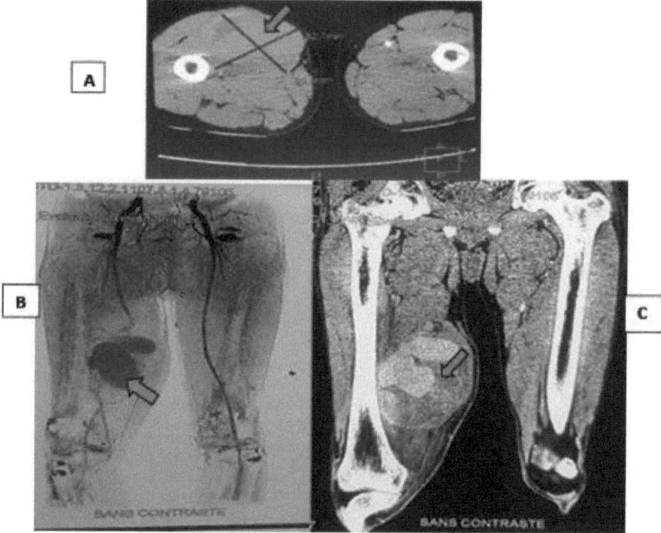

Figure 59: A, B, C. False aneurysm of the right superficial femoral artery (Andre FESTOC Centre, CHU-ME Bamako).

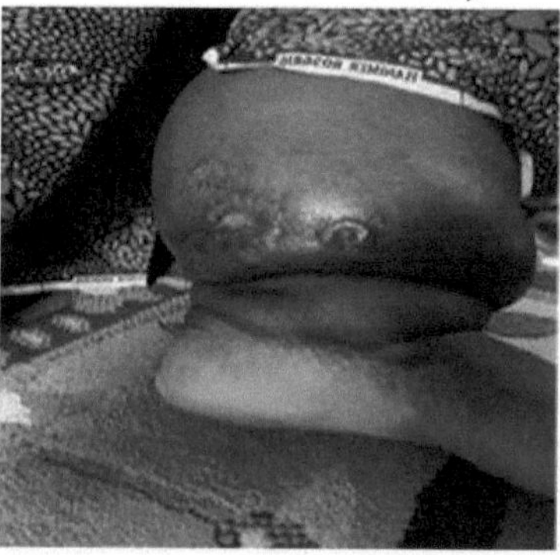

Figure 60: Superinfected lymphoedema of the MIG. (Andre FESTOC Centre, CHU-ME, Bamako).

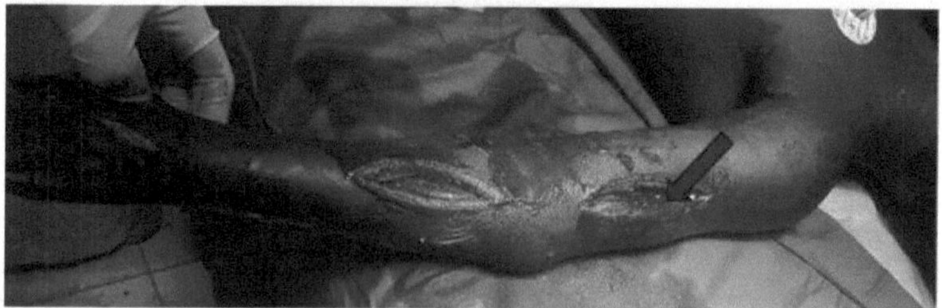

Figure 61: *MSG aponeurotomy* in an 8-year-old child (Andre FESTOC Centre, CHU-ME, Bamako).

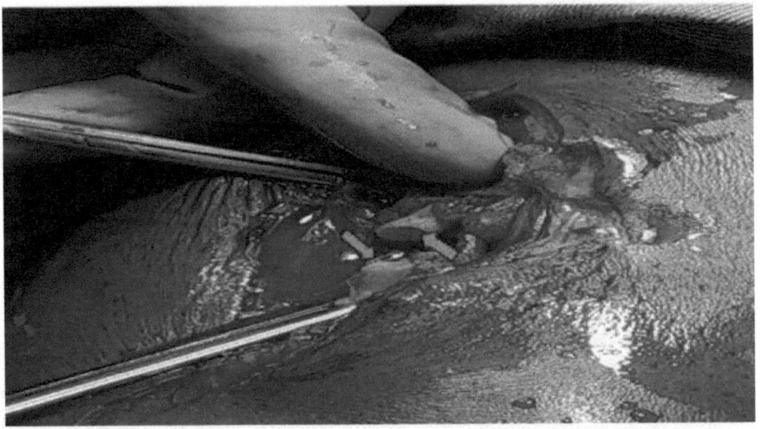

Figure 62: Complete section of the left humeral artery following ballistic trauma (Andre FESTOC Centre, CHU-ME, Bamako).

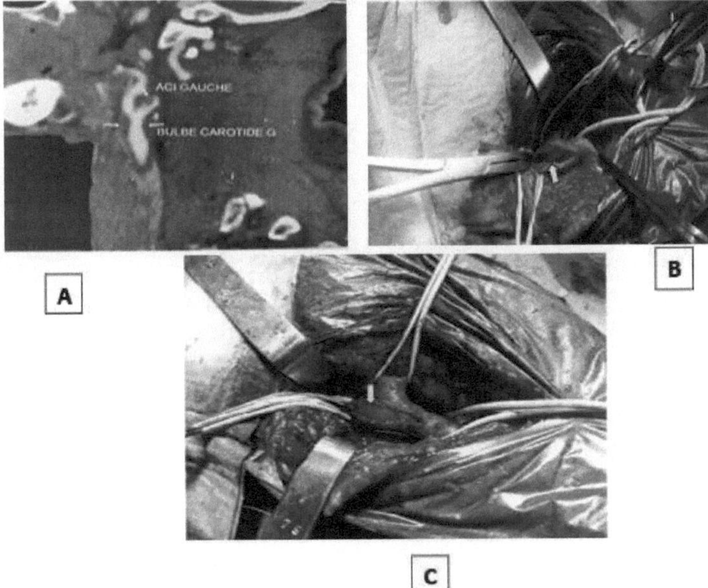

Figure 63: A. Occlusion of the left internal carotid artery, B. Endarterectomy of the tripod of the left carotid artery, **C**. Patch for closure of the endarterectomy of the tripod of the left carotid artery (Centre André FESTOC CHU-ME, Bamako).

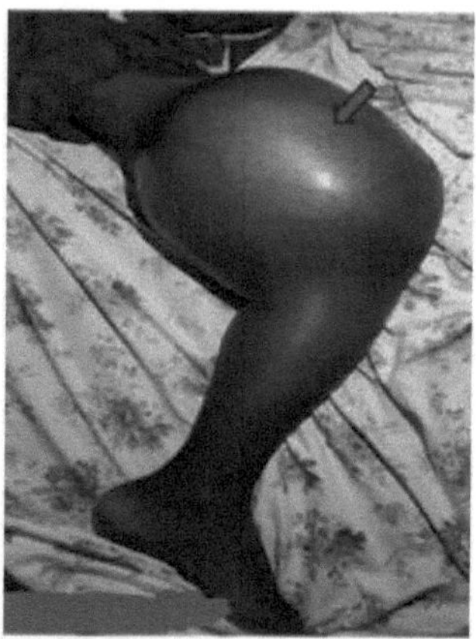

Figure 64: Osteosarcoma of the left thigh (André FESTOC Centre, CHU-ME, Bamako).

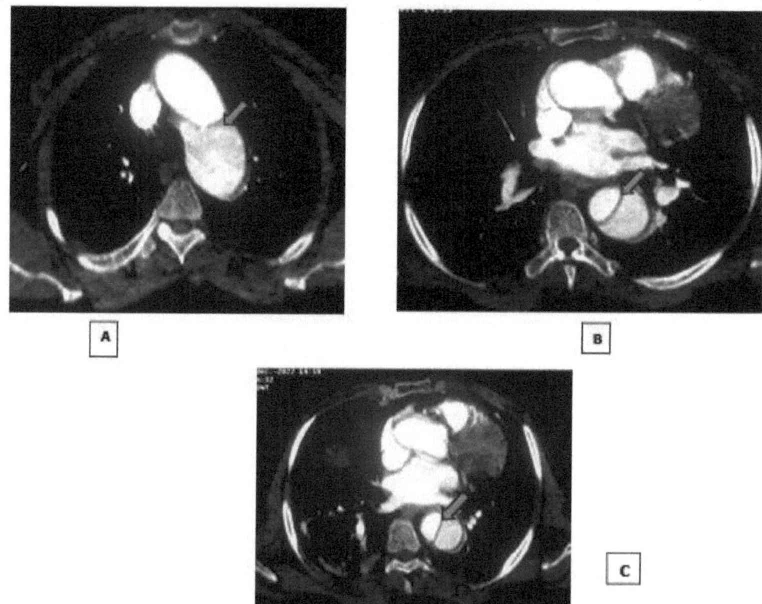

Figure 65: A, B, C. Axial sections of thoracic angioscanner showing a type A aortic dissection. (Andre FESTOC Centre, CHU-ME Bamako).

APPENDICES

Investigation form I. <u>Patient no.</u>: 1. <u>identity</u>

IP : .... Last name: .... First name: ....

DOB: .../.../...Sex: ..... Blood type:............. Residence: .... Profession: .... N° tel
: Provenance : 1 CScom : 2 CSREF : 3 Hôpital régional : 4 CHU : 5 Clinique privée : 6
Lui-même :

2.   Date of consultation: .... 3. <u>Reason for consultation</u>: Thoracic surgery :
Chest pain: 1.../yes 2.../no Chest deformity: 1.../yes 2.../no Dyspnoea: 1.../yes 2.../no -
Pleural effusion: Pleurisy: 1.../yes 2.../no haemothorax: 1.../yes 2.../no pyothorax: 1.../yes
2.../no pneumothorax: 1.../yes 2.../no Effusion: 1.../yes 2.../no. - Pericardial effusion:
1.../yes 2.../no - Chest trauma: Closed: 1.../yes 2.../no Open: 1.../yes 2.../yes - Thoracic
tumour: 1.../yes 2.../no 3.../intra 4.../extra 5.../linear 6.../malignant Location: 1.../primary
2.../secondary - Tuberculosis: 1...yes 2.../no sequelae: 1.../yes 2.../no

- Others :

Vascular surgery

- Plantar tingling: 1.../yes 2.../no - Walking perimeter: 1.../ ≤ 100m 2.../ ≤ 500m - Arterial
ischaemia: 1.../yes 2.../no location: - DVT: 1.../yes 2.../no location: - Diabetic foot: 1.../yes
2.../no location: - Varicose veins: 1.../yes 2.../no 3.../VGS 4.../VPS 5.../right 6.../left
7.../Varicose ulcer - Lymphoedema: 1.../yes 2.../no location: - Arterial aneurysm: 1.../yes
2.../no location: - Aortic aneurysm: 1.../yes 2.../no location: - Carotid stenosis: 1.../yes 2.../no
location: - AVF: 1.../yes 2.../no 3.../left 4.../right 5.../proximal 6.../dislateral

II. <u>History of the disease</u> :

. start: . progress: . diagnosis :

III. <u>Background</u> :

Medical: Surgical: Gynaecological :

IV. <u>Physical examinations</u> :

Pathological organ: .   General signs: .   General condition:/good....../poor....... Weight :
......kg Height : ......cm

. conjunctivae:/normo - coloured....../pales....... .   Femoral pulses perceived:/yes....../no........ .
Heart rate: ......batt/min .   Respiratory rate: ......cycle/min .   Oxygen saturation: ....% .
Blood pressure: ....mmhg

Inspection:

.   Chest deformity: 1.../or 2.../no .   Jugular turgidity: 1.../yes 2.../no .   Collateral venous
circulation:1.../yes 2.../no .   Signs of struggle: 1.../yes 2.../no .   Associated malformations:
1.../yes 2.../no

. palpation

.   Normal peak shock: 1.../yes 2.../no .   Tremor:1.../yes 2.../no .   Auscultation: .
Cardiac :

. BDC: audible:1.../yes 2.../no regular: 1.../yes 2.../no .   Systolic murmur: 1.../yes 2..../non
. If yes, specify location: 0..../mitral 2.../pulmonary 3.../aortic 4.../tricuspid .   Diastolic
murmur: 1.../yes 2..../no. . If yes, specify focus: 0.../mitral 2.../ pulmonary 3.../aortic
4.../tricuspid .   Continuous murmur:1.../yes 2..../no
. If yes, specify focus: 0.../mitral 2.../pulmonary 3.../aortic 4.../tricuspid
. muffled: 1.../yes 2..../no .   Gallop: 1/yes 2..../no .   Tachycardia: 1.../yes 2...../non .
Bradycardia: 1.../yes 2..../non .   Pulmonary: .   Vesicular murmur: 1.../yes 2.../no .

Vocal vibration: 1.../yes 2..../no .   Crackling rales: 1/yes 2..../no .   Sibilants: 1/yes 2.../no .   Abdominal examination: . General appearance of abdomen: soft: 1.../yes 2.../no distended: 1...yes 2.../no CVC: 1.../yes 2.../no .   Hepatomegaly: 1.../yes 2..../non . Splenomegaly:1.../yes 2..../non .   Mass: 1.../yes 2..../non .   Elsewhere: other to report: 1..../yes 2..../no specified :.............

V. <u>Paraclinical examinations</u>: a. Front chest X-ray :

Quality criteria met: 1.../yes 2.../no Container: normal: 1..../yes 2.../no if not, please specify:....................

Container:

Cardio - thoracic index: 1.../normal 2.../ cardiomegaly Cardiac silhouette: 1.../ situs solitus 2.../situs invertus

Lung parenchyma: 1.../normal 2.../hypovascular 3.../hypervascular Pleural effusion: 1.../liquid 2.../pneumatic 3.../mixed Mass: 1.../intrathoracic 2.../extrathoracic

b. <u>Electrocardiography</u> :

. frequency:1.../normal 2.../tachycardia 3..../bradycardia . rhythm: sinus 1..../yes 2.. 3.../regular 4.../irregular . axis: 1.../normal 2..../anormal .   P-R: normal: 1.../yes 2.../no BAV 1= 1.../yes 2.../no Mobitz: 1.../yes I 2 .../yes II 3.../no BAV3: 1.../yes 2.../no

. hypertrophy:1.../yes 2.../no atrial: 1...yes 2.../no ventricular: 1.../yes 2.../no

. atrial fibrillation: 1.../yes 2.../no ventricular fibrillation: /1...yes 2.../no . right bundle branch block: 1.../yes 2.../no left bundle branch block:1.../yes 2.../no hemi block: 1.../yes 2.../no . signs of ischemia: 1.../yes 2...../non Other to be specified: ....

c. <u>Cardiac ultrasound</u> :

Ao: mm OG: mm VGd: mm VGs: mm FEVG: % FR: %

Valvulopathies: 1..../aortic 2.../ pulmonary 3.../tricuspid 4..../mitral Dry pericardium: 1.../yes 2.../no Other to be specified: ....

d. <u>Thoracic angioscan</u> :

1.../done 2.../no 3..../Result

<u>Angioscan of the upper limbs</u> :

Calcifications: 1.../yes 2..../no 3.../ Location: Stenosis: 1.../yes 3.../no 3.../ Location: Ischaemia: 1.../yes 2.../no 3... Location:

<u>Angioscan of the lower limbs</u> :

Calcifications: 1.../yes 2..../no 3.../ Location Stenosis: 1.../yes 3.../no 3.../ Location Ischaemia: 1.../yes 2.../no 3... Location

e. <u>Biology</u> :

.   White blood cells: ....10 mm/3 predominantly hyperleukocytosis:.............. .   Red blood cells: ....10mm/6 .   Haemoglobin: ....g/dl Haematocrit: ....% VGM:................fl CCMH:...............g/dl .   CRP: ....mg/dl .   Blood glucose: ....mg/dl . Urea: ....mmol/L .   Creatin : ....umol/l . TP: ....%

.   TCK : ....

.   HIV serology:1...//positive 2.../negative .   HBsAg: 1.../positive 2..../negative . AcHbc: 1.../positive 2..../negative .   Emmel test: 1.../positive 2.../negative . ECBC: 1.../yes 2.../no Appearance of fluid: 1.../Hematic 2.../transuda 3.../exsuda Germs isolated: 1.../yes 2.../no 3...: to be specified: antibiogram: 1.../yes 2.../no

. ANAPATH : 1.../yes 2.../no 3.../linear 4.../unlinear 5.../to be specified :........

.   Xpert gene: 1.../yes 2.../no MBT: 1.../yes 2.../no

f. <u>Medical treatments</u>:

Hypertension: 1....yes 2.../no .   Diuretic:1.../yes 2..../non .   ACE inhibitor: 1.../yes 2..../no
.   Beta-blocker: 1.../yes 2..../no. .   Diabetes: 1.../yes 2.../no 3.../insulin therapy 4.../ADO
.   Anticoagulant: 1.../yes 2...../non . Antibiotic: 1.../yes 2....../non .   Analgesic: 1.../yes
2.../no

g. <u>Surgical treatment</u> :

Age at time of surgery................

Weight at time of surgery: ....kg Height at time of surgery: ....cm Thoracic surgery: 1.../open 2.../closed Plastic surgery: 1.../yes 2.../no

Infection surgery: 1.../yes 2.../no Trauma surgery: 1.../yes 2.../no Vascular surgery: Ischaemic pathology due to : 1.../embolism 2.../arthritis Vascular trauma: 1.../yes 2.../no Vascular malformation: 1.../yes 2.../no Aneurysm: 1.../yes 2.../no Diabetic foot: 1.../yes 2.../no Orthopaedic treatment: 1.../yes 2.../no Physiotherapy treatment: 1.../yes 2.../no

VI. <u>Development</u> :

a. Immediate post-operative complications: 1.../yes 2..../no .   3.../bleeding 4.../ischaemia 5.../ thrombosis b.   Late post-operative complications: 1.../yes 2..../no 3.../If yes, please specify **c.** Post-operative follow-up: 1.../regular 2.../irregular 3.../lost sight **e. Rehospitalisation:** 1.../Yes 2..../No 3.../If yes, please specify 4.../Reason 5.../Duration 6..../Exeat 7..../Deceased

Information sheet

Name: TANGARA

First name: Souleymane

Title of thesis: Clinical and therapeutic aspects of thoracic and vascular pathologies at the Andre FESTOC centre of the CHU Mere - Enfant le " Luxembourg " in Bamako (Mali).

Year of defence : 2024

City of defence: Bamako (Mali)

Nationality: Malian

Depository: Library of the Faculty of Medicine, Pharmacy and Odontostomatology du Mali (F.M.P.O.S).

Sector of interest: Thoracic and vascular surgery.

Email : Tangara8a@gmail.com, **Tel :** +22377696755

Resume

Introduction: Thoracic and vascular surgery has been practised for centuries. The practice of thoracic and vascular surgery in Mali dates back to the first years after independence (1960). We initiated this work to study the epidemiological, clinical and therapeutic aspects of thoracic and vascular pathologies at the Andre FESTOC Centre of the CHU Mere - Enfant le " Luxembourg " in Bamako (Mali).

Methodology: This was a retrospective, descriptive study carried out at the Andre FESTOC Centre of the Mere Enfant "Luxembourg" Hospital in Bamako, from 01 January 2018 to 31 December 2022. It focused on the records of operated and non-operated patients treated for thoracic and vascular surgery.

Results: We enrolled 1720 patients, 581 of whom were managed for thoracic surgery and 1139 for vascular surgery. A total of 792 patients were operated on, i.e. 46.04% of patients managed. Non-operated patients either benefited from medical treatment or other non-invasive treatments.

The overall mean age of the patients was 51.34 years, with a standard deviation of 19.51 and extremes of 2 months and 123 years, all of whom were adults. Only 76 patients were under 15 years of age, representing 4.45% of all patients. The sex ratio was 0.9, with housewives accounting for the highest proportion (41.51%). Overall hospital mortality was 5.93%.

Conclusion: Thoracic and vascular surgery has developed rapidly over the last two decades in Mali and is now routinely performed with reliable and reproducible results. However, minimally invasive techniques (thoracoscopy and endovascular surgery) need to be popularised.

Key words: epidemiological and therapeutic aspects, thoracic and vascular pathology, Andre FESTOC centre, Mali.

Hippocratic Oath

In the presence of the masters of this faculty, my dear fellow students, in front of the effigy of Hippocrates,

I promise and swear, in the name of the supreme being, to be faithful to the laws of honour and probity in the practice of medicine.

I will give my care free of charge to the needy and will never demand a salary above my work, nor will I take part in any clandestine sharing of fees.

If I am allowed inside houses, my eyes will not see what goes on there, my tongue will keep silent about the secrets entrusted to me, and my status will not be used to corrupt people or encourage crime.

I will not allow considerations of religion, nation, race, party or social class to come between my duty and my patient.

I will maintain absolute respect for human life from the moment of conception. Even under threat, I will not allow my medical knowledge to be used against the law of humanity.

Respectful and grateful to my teachers, I will give back to their children the education I received from their fathers.

May men esteem me, if I am faithful to my promises

May I be shamed and despised by my colleagues if I fail to do so.

I swear it.

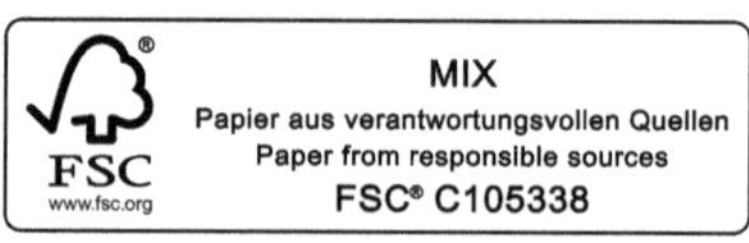

Printed by Books on Demand GmbH, Norderstedt / Germany